DEEP IN THE BRAIN

Helmut Dubiel

DEEP IN THE BRAIN

*Translated from the German
by Philip Schmitz*

Europa
editions

Europa Editions
116 East 16th Street
New York, N.Y. 10003
www.europaeditions.com
info@europaeditions.com

Library of Congress Cataloging in Publication Data is available
ISBN 978-1-933372-70-9

Dubiel, Helmut
Deep In the Brain

The translation of this work was supported
by a grant from the Goethe-Institut
which is funded by the German Ministry of Foreign Affairs

Book design by Emanuele Ragnisco
www.mekkanografici.com

Cover illustration: Arthur Menton, *A Symbolic Head*, 1879

Prepress by Plan.ed – Rome

Printed in Canada

CONTENTS

DEEP IN THE BRAIN

for Hella Becker

PROLOGUE

From the Wetterau rest stop the Taunus drops off sharply toward the south. When the sky is cloudy or overcast, the reflection of the lights of Frankfurt can already be seen early in the evening. The glare of the oncoming headlights blurs with the faraway lights of the city in the smeary film the windshield wipers leave behind. I'm driving slowly in the right lane, stuck between two trucks from Poland. I take my hands off the wheel. A passage from di Lampedusa's *The Leopard* comes to mind in which the Prince contemplates those moments of his life he would like to relive when he faces death. I have recalled these lines so often that they have blazed a trail of dreams into my sleep. Lately, of course, the memory is tinged with alienation. I'm disturbed by the briefness of the time that the Prince would like to relive if he were given the opportunity. And his choice of wishes bothers me. He wants to relive only his unequivocally happy minutes: for example, the moment he awaits his bride on a flower-scented bed of love.

As a petty bourgeois perhaps I am less choosy than the Prince. I am also the contemporary of an age in which people have learned that everything has its two sides. For me, there is simply more that comes to mind: my arrival in New York as a dishwasher on board the passenger liner

Europa in the late 1960s. In those days the structural work on the World Trade Center had just been completed, and the twin towers came into view in the early morning fog. The sight of the active Kilauea Volcano in Hawaii by night. The Iguazu Waterfalls, the endless roads of Patagonia, the sight of the stars over Sinai in the 1970s. The irrepressible happiness in the face of my son when I would pick him up at kindergarten in Florence in the late 1980s. The joy—it is difficult to describe—of experiencing how a text created at my desk is read and discussed by many people. And, not to be forgotten, love.

Evidently, it is not only the number of my moments of happiness that distinguishes me from the Prince. In his life the good and the bad, beauty and horror, were clearly distinct from one another. In my life, however, happy and unhappy developments do not unfold in parallel, with no connection, but are instead superimposed on each other, forming what are often bizarre patterns. For example, when I think back to those days in New York, as a dishwasher on the old Europa, I cannot help thinking about that eleventh day of September in 2001 when I watched from a rooftop in Brooklyn as the two towers collapsed. In a similar way the experience of love and commitment in my life is knotted together with a sense of fear and guilt, betrayal and infidelity, with memories of my wrongdoings against others and theirs against me.

I'm sick. Remembering the beginning and the course of the illness brings my trail of dreams to an end. When I arrive at that point, a sleepless night lies ahead of me. Fifteen years ago I "had" the disease the way other people have diabetes or osteoarthritis. Today, as ever fewer people are capable of differentiating between the disease and me personally, the disease has me. It inundates me with inter-fering signals, the fluctuating effects of the medications with their constraints and incessant agitation. Initially, this identification with my illness has to do with its incurabili-ty, and then with the fact that it impairs the very physical communicative competencies that people employ to estab-lish relationships with others.

Nevertheless, given the choice between living in the body and mind of some other (healthy) person and con-tinuing life within my own, I wouldn't hesitate for a sec-ond to decide in favor of myself.

I was startled by an earsplitting horn that was blowing as loud as a ship's siren. My car had drifted into the mid-dle lane and a truck was bearing down on me at high speed from behind. There was a harsh crack. Only after the truck disappeared into the night honking furiously, did I notice that my side mirror had been torn off.

I n an atlas of neurology the various provinces of the brain are represented in much the same way as the regions of the earth on a geographical map. Deep within the brain, about where the cerebrum tapers into the brain stem, we find the so-called substantia nigra, the "black substance." Leading from the "black substance" to a neighboring area called the striatum is a narrow band of tissue only a few centimeters long. The striatum is the home of dopamine, one of the brain's messenger chemicals that is responsible in the human building plan for controlling and coordinating the body's musculoskeletal system. This region of the brain, which is no larger than a walnut, controls the infinitely complicated interplay of the muscle groups that is required, for example, for a person with an awareness of her own dignity to stride vigorously and elegantly through a ballroom. Much the same as the showman in a pedestrian zone, who becomes rigid like a statue, is only able to perform by virtue of the neuromuscular control required to coordinate the ever-changing sequence of excitatory and inhibitory impulses.

Parkinson's disease (PD) attacks predominantly older people between the ages of fifty-five and sixty-five. The probability of developing the disease increases with age. Epidemiologists, those who study the spread and prevalence of diseases, use the following rule of thumb: Parkinson's occurs in roughly one percent of those over sixty, two percent of those over seventy, and so on. In more precise terms, Parkinson's occurs in close to 0.16 percent of the total population, striking 16 out of every 10,000 people. Accordingly, Parkinson's is considered a "disease of the elderly."

I was forty-six years old when I was diagnosed with the illness, which makes me a case of "young onset Parkinson's," or YOP. It is often alleged that the age of onset is dropping. In other words, people are supposedly falling ill at an increasingly young age. It is difficult to obtain statistics about this. The growing number of cases diagnosed under the age of forty-five, and even under forty, could just as easily be the result of improved diagnostic techniques. Moreover, people who fall ill at an early age get a lot of public attention, so that mass-media awareness of Parkinson's disease has increased.

The causes of Parkinson's are unknown. The many promises of brain researchers notwithstanding, a scientific breakthrough which would explain PD and provide a cure has as yet failed to materialize. There is good evidence to suggest that the discovery of the causes and perhaps even a cure may emerge from the partial results of the molecular puzzle that are currently being compiled with great energy.

Another reason Parkinson's is viewed as a disease of the elderly is that its symptoms are embedded in the unspecific motor disturbances that almost everyone develops at an advanced age. A general stiffening of the muscles, a certain rigidity of movement, and a slight tremor are by themselves not symptomatic of an illness. However, to state that a mild case of Parkinson's manifests itself in almost every aging process would be to trivialize the matter. One might say that the aging process derails. In Parkinson's, they say, the substantia nigra "dies."

The signs of the disease do not present themselves with empirical precision. PD can be masked in nonspecific back pain or depression for many years. In the end, a diagnosis is based on the traditionally observed motor disturbances as well as an interpretive evaluation of the symptoms within the individual's life cycle. The final piece of information has only become available through the latest medical technology. By using a radioactive contrast medium and so-called "positron emission tomography," low activity in specific areas of the brain can be imaged with absolute certainty. But the procedure is expensive and is only administered in ambiguous cases. Generally, the specific quality of the motor disturbances and the patient's response to L-dopa, the first-line medication, will allow a sufficiently precise diagnosis.

In Parkinson's disease, named after its discoverer James Parkinson, the tissue that produces dopamine dies at a faster rate than corresponds to the normal aging process. Naturally, the problem is not the lack of dopamine alone, but rather the imbalance it causes in other messenger chemicals such as acetylcholine, noradrenalin, serotonin, etc.

The illness does not affect gross motor skills alone, but rather the entire musculature. For example, no area of the body has more muscles than the face. Thus, a pathological deficiency of the messenger chemical dopamine impairs not only the movement of the trunk musculature but also the entire range of a person's individual self-expression.

Human beings are more than just animated machines; they communicate not only through speech but with their entire body. One of the unmistakable signs of this disease is the appearance of a frozen facial expression or even the occasional involuntary grimace. This often has dire consequences for the social acceptance of Parkinson's sufferers. What the professional views as a symptom that can be compared objectively to the symptoms of other patients, the layperson construes as a bizarre trait of a particular individual. People who can no longer control their facial expression can also no longer reckon with the average person's willingness to distinguish between the disease and its victim. There are moving accounts of Parkinson's sufferers who gradually went to pieces because people, their colleagues at work, who did not know of their illness, derided them as drunkards, imbeciles and malingerers.

The symptoms that identify Parkinson's and play a major role in traditional diagnosis are divided into tremor, rigor and akinesia. "Tremor" refers to the hands shaking in a resting position, "rigor" to the stiffening of the entire body's musculature, and akinesia to the poverty of all body movement. In the early stages the distribution and severity of all these symptoms are still highly individual. There are patients who suffer visibly only from tremor. Another type of patient exhibits primarily the symptoms of hyperkinesias and rigidity. As the years wear on, however, the nature of the symptoms becomes more uniform, so that one might have the impression that the patients are all related to one another. Only a small amount of training is required to recognize full-blown Parkinson's in everyday life. Patients stand in a slightly forward-flexed posture as if they were about to fall over. Their eyes look down at the ground. There is a poverty of facial expression. To the healthy observer, their body seems to signal a frightened submissiveness.

From the perspective of the victim, it is a particularly depressing fact that the first symptoms only emerge when more than half of the substantia nigra has already been damaged. When the first tremor appears, when one often stumbles or stutters, when one's left arm hangs down from the shoulder joint with so little swing that an automatic wristwatch will no longer wind by itself, it's already too late. But speaking of "too late" draws a false analogy to illnesses where an early diagnosis still holds out the promise of a cure. For PD there is as yet no such cure. Nevertheless, all of the advice books, especially those written by physicians, recommend early diagnosis because it creates greater flexibility for prescribing individually tailored medications. Naturally, this advantage must be offset against the disadvantage of early knowledge. It is, after all, best to know of an inescapable fate as late as possible.

The so-called "gold standard" in drug therapy is L-dopa. A material that is converted into natural dopamine inside the brain, L-dopa utilizes the ability of nerve cells to produce dopamine far above their natural capacity, at least for a time. After a certain period, called "the honeymoon" by neurologists with romantic irony, almost all patients develop side effects. These are large involuntary movements, and in the end it becomes altogether impossible to say whether they are a direct result of the disease or of the medication. During those last years there were days when I was easily swallowing up to thirty pills. Of course, I wasn't taking each of the pills according to my symptomatic needs but was following a medication regimen determined at the time by the neurologist who was treating me. Being dependent upon medications to that degree is a torture, a kind of medically prescribed drug addiction. The myriad pills must be taken in a certain sequence. Deviate from the path, either deliberately or inadvertently, and punishment swiftly follows. If the organism is undersupplied, it lapses into an "off period," causing a rigidity that affects the entire musculature and can be very painful. In the event of an accidental overdose, the organism succumbs to disruptive, socially conspicuous dyskinesias and agitation.

There are a considerable number of new medications that are usually geared to complementing the shortcomings of L-dopa, the so-called "agonists." These are pills which are effective against the core symptoms of Parkinson's. As time goes on, every patient suffers from additional symptoms arising only indirectly from the disease. Many suffer from constipation, swallowing disturbances, speech disorders, back pain, depression, insomnia, etc., which are also treated with medications. The entire regimen is crowned with medication for the gastrointestinal problems one might expect as a result of the excessive medication intake.

At present, the pharmaceutical treatment strategy is still dominant, but for about ten years a new surgical procedure called deep brain stimulation (DBS) has been practiced. If only for financial reasons, this surgical technique will never have the same impact as drug therapy. According to current medical research, only fifteen percent of Parkinson's patients are candidates. Deep brain stimulation involves sending weak electrical signals to the affected regions of the brain by means of a pacemaker implanted in the body. The fact remains, however, that neither the pharmaceutical approach nor the surgical procedure—their great efficacy notwithstanding—alter the underlying degenerative pathology of the tissue in the substantia nigra. They alleviate the consequences of the degeneration, but they do not cure it.

One of my many inklings that I was afflicted with Parkinson's came in the early 1990s. It was the most beautiful day of my life to date. In late May I had driven from Vienna to Lake Neusiedl with Corinna, who at the time embodied the promise of a great love for me. I still vividly remember our room, the clatter of the breakfast dishes in the small bed-and-breakfast, and the curtain in front of the window billowing in the summer breeze. We made love. At the climax I trembled over my entire body. For several seconds my left hand took on a life of its own and made erratic, chaotic movements. I explained these symptoms, to myself and my lover, as the result of my inordinate passion. And maybe this interpretation was not incorrect. In spite of its bizarre dimensions I failed to take this symptomatic event seriously because it occurred within the beautiful context of love.

From then on symptoms began to appear at increasingly short intervals. In retrospect they fit together to form a clear trail. As a part of my everyday experience, though, they were difficult to interpret. There were bothersome sensations that manifested in both mental and physical form. There was an almost constant feeling of stiffness, roughly comparable in degree to the loss of agility and flexibility that healthy people experience after a day of skiing if they are not conditioned. In addition, there was a slight tremor when my hands were in a resting position, which was barely noticeable. Dizziness, which I dismissed as a circulatory problem, was rare. As time progressed, I had a growing, fundamental sense that I was no longer in control of my movements. I felt like a worn out car where the steering responds very imprecisely and only after a number of seconds.

The panic attacks were the worst. The first of them, which I can still remember exactly, befell me at the airport in Pisa. I was in the waiting room after having my hand luggage checked, when I suddenly had the impression that the ceiling was being pressed down toward the floor by a gigantic vise, and that it was threatening to crush me. At the same time, something told me that it must be an illusion because my fellow passengers were evidently noticing nothing of the kind. I, however, was struck from one moment to the next by diarrhea, difficulty breathing, shaky knees, chest pain, and sweaty hands.

Only in retrospect was I inclined to see in this first panic attack a causal connection with a minor incident that had occurred immediately beforehand. The waiting room was sectioned off from the apron of the airport by a plate glass wall. Suddenly, in a group of passengers heading for their airplane on the other side of the plate glass, I recognized an Italian woman whom I knew in passing. She had once been my language teacher, and my memories of her were not pleasant. She had poked fun at my Teutonic stiffness. I now drew attention to myself by waving my hand in a choppy motion I perceived as typically Italian. She separated herself from the group along with her partner, laughingly pointed me out to him, and then repeated my choppy hand motion with openly sarcastic intentions. Her mimicry of my gesture immediately made it clear to me that from the perspective of an external observer my expressive behavior was already a far cry from the internal image that I, like everyone else, carried of myself. My actual expressions were no more than a caricatured, distorted representation of their underlying intentions.

I was and continue to be a university professor, and at the time I had a large circle of acquaintances, colleagues and friends. In addition, I was the father of a boy who was entering elementary school during the period I am describing. The very day-to-day responsibilities, tasks and activities of daily life such as driving a car—especially chauffeuring children—teaching students, not to mention giving lectures, became a source of harrowing anxiety attacks. And yet it took several years before I was even able to interpret the various physical indications such as stomach ache, shaky knees, a tendency to diarrhea and racing heart as signs of anxiety and panic. All of these conditions, together with almost constant fatigue and diffuse pain in my limbs, made it clear to me that something was fundamentally wrong. When my very first symptoms appeared, I would still discuss them with several confidential, generally male, friends. But they were as clueless as I. It was precisely the parallelism of physical and psychiatric symptoms that was so confusing. The more they coalesced into a neurological picture, the more I kept silent about them.

I was so distraught because in those days, early in the last decade of the twentieth century, I still believed that it was possible to achieve happiness not just momentarily but as a condition, so to speak. It wasn't my bitter but as yet abstract premonition of being gravely ill that clearly demonstrated how illusory this expectation was. Rather, it was experiencing the diverse fears, the daily impairment of my lifestyle and the constant, inexplicable exhaustion after performing tasks that had once been a source of joy, that permanently darkened my horizon. The Matthew principle also applies to those who have been saddened: misfortune is heaped on the unfortunate.

Corinna from Vienna, whom I thought I loved more than anything else at the time, could no longer endure the hiding game she was playing with her partner, who had turned mistrustful. The mountain of lies that our love was built upon stifled the magic of our nights. She hadn't said anything, but we both knew, and each of us was aware that the other one knew, that our farewell at Vienna Western Station in June would be the last time we met. I had a foreboding that the short happy spell was only to be an incubation period for an unhappiness that would last until my death. I suddenly recalled insights that had once been at the forefront of my mind. The realization, for example, that one can only achieve happiness or even contentment through one's own effort, and that the inclination to borrow expectations of happiness against a romantic attachment will destroy the happiness over the long term.

I learned only later through studying clinical accounts and the experience reports of patients that the outbreak of dramatic, chronic and especially neurological diseases is often accompanied by nonspecific psychophysical states of exhaustion. The fact that serious diseases often use psychophysical breakdowns as a Trojan horse may mislead one into interpreting the underlying disease process in a simple, psychosomatic sense. To me, the hypothesis of an emotional immune system would appear more fitting. In addition to an intact physical immune system, every person who is physically and mentally well enough also possesses an emotional immune system, The latter can be so weakened by numerous traumatic stressors that it collapses, resulting in the manifestation of a pathology which was long present in a latent, germinal form.

I was already standing on the lowest step of the Vienna–Amsterdam night train which was cleared for departure. At that moment, time stood still, and I mean literally. At the minute the train was scheduled to leave, some esoteric defect for which there would also be no comprehensible official explanation later on, paralyzed all of the clocks in Vienna Western Station.

But this wonder only impressed the train engineer for several minutes. Our love had been strong enough to stop the clocks in the station but not the train, the further course of events, or time itself. When I arrived in Frankfurt the next morning, shattered and poorly rested, my legs buckled underneath me on the platform. The emergency doctor had me admitted to a hospital for a neurological examination.

That same morning an intake interview was conducted at the Frankfurt University Clinic; I recall only fragments of this. The admitting physician was a young and apparently newly licensed doctor who limited himself for the most part to reading off questions from pre-printed materials. He recorded my answers with scrupulous care on a notepad adorned with the familiar Goethe logo of Frankfurt University. When he came to the questions about hereditary diseases in the family, he inquired specifically and in detail regarding any occurrence of Parkinson's. I had read enough about neurological diseases in the meantime to understand that the question he posed with such determination actually already represented the answer to the only question that worried me. For about a year I had been making a habit of browsing medical dictionaries in bookstores, libraries, and the relevant sections of department stores. Just the day before, I had come across a popular introduction to neurological diseases in a Viennese bookstore. My hands were shaking as I replaced the book on the shelf after reading an exact description of my symptoms under the rubric of Parkinson's Disease.

I immediately broke out in tears and started talking some kind of nonsense about my young girlfriend in Vienna, simply to show the young man the vastness of my despair. I told him that if his question was meant to imply that I suffered from the disease, he was wrong. After all, I was well informed about the symptomatology of Parkinson's. As I struggled to regain my composure, I told him that several months before, on the advice of my orthopedist, I had consulted a neurologist in private practice who found nothing. Of course, that was only partially true. The whole truth was that the neurologist found extremely poor nerve conduction in the left side of the body three times in succession—a finding which, as I later learned, is an indication of Parkinson's. The neurologist had terminated the examination because he believed that the consistently extremely low readings were a sign that his equipment was defective. But perhaps he was also simply a sagacious man who wanted to spare me the truth for just a little while longer. Today, it seems more likely to me that he in fact knew exactly what the low nerve conduction results indicated. But even neurologists can show sensitivity. He didn't want to spoil the weekend, not only for me but also for himself.

The young neurologist at the Frankfurt University Clinic was an entirely different story. The as yet unspoken diagnosis seemed to give him sadistic pleasure. He told me rudely with unconcealed disgust that I should pull myself together. My daring challenge to his authority had the effect of really infuriating him. He referred to a previous skull x-ray that clearly showed shrinkage of my brain mass. Radiologists to whom I later showed the x-ray assured me that the finding of reduced brain mass was in general thoroughly unscientific, and that in my specific case it was nonsense. Seen through the eyes of an impartial third party, our mutual inability to deal with the situation must have looked very funny. The resident physician, who was extremely aggravated, resorted to a white lie as an elegant means to escape the painful embarrassment. He would not presume to diagnose my illness. He avoided the term Parkinson's. His questions were solely directed at excluding the possibility that I was suffering from a brain tumor, or multiple sclerosis, or a silent stroke. The actual determination of my condition would be the prerogative of the head physician.

The white-haired, suntanned head physician had apparently been alerted by his assistant and sacrificed his lunch hour to diagnose me then and there. As we walked to his office, he observed my weary, shuffling gait with professional curiosity. His enjoyment of his own professional elegance was apparent as he examined my limited mobility. My feelings toward him consisted of collegial sympathy and admiration at the same time. He reminded me of myself, striding peripatetically back and forth, through a lecture hall, publicly dwelling on my thoughts. When he asked me to use my left hand and imitate a person screwing in a light bulb, all I could produce was a helpless tremor. Even a gentle push on the shoulder to test my equilibrium threw me completely off balance. I was incapable of touching the tip of my nose with my index finger on the first attempt. "My younger colleague was correct," he said. "You are suffering from Parkinson's disease beyond any doubt." He dismissed my request that he at least take a look at the x-ray, pointing out that in cases of Parkinson's x-ray images are diagnostically inconclusive.

2.

Theories, models, and concepts are not simply the toys of scientists. They also play an important role in the everyday lives of laypeople—for example, in the way humans experience their bodies. This applies in two respects. First, they bring order into chaos. A new concept, a new theory, will occasionally help to shape a Gestalt out of data and sensations that up to that point had formed only a diffuse conglomeration. One might ask, therefore, whether the symptoms of Parkinson's existed before there was a name for them.

Once the term Parkinson's had been introduced into my world, most notably the constant fatigue and anxiety attacks could no longer be dismissed as the hypochondriac symptoms of a severe neurotic. The diagnosis brought order into an apparently random series of symptoms, just as one creates order in randomly scattered iron filings simply by passing a magnet over them at close range. With respect to the dimension of time, the diagnosis had the paradoxical effect of being both disquieting and quieting. On the one hand, it marked the starting point of a state of separation from other people, the irrevocable onset of exclusion from the circle of those who are (apparently still) "healthy" and "normal." On the other hand, due to the chaotic multiplicity of the symptoms, the diagnosis was a kind of black box where one could deposit every symptom, every form of discomfort. The headaches and back pain that plagued my life until then to a greater or lesser degree, ceased the day I accepted the diagnosis. I also no longer perceived my mood swings, depressive episodes, shuddering, limb pain, and other flu-like symptoms in and of themselves, but rather as respective instances of unsuccessful Parkinson's management. Thus, in one sense, life's brutal randomness manifested itself in the diagnosis. In another sense, the diagnosis marked the beginning of a new regime of order in which things ceased to appear coincidental.

At the beginning of the illness I consulted a large number of doctors. They differed from one another in the adeptness with which they introduced me to coping with the disease. In the long run, the ones I experienced as trustworthy—totally irrespective of whether they were neurologists or general practitioners—were always those who would not support my childlike desire for order, predictability, and a lack of ambiguity, and were simply able to admit how little they really knew. My experiences with this kind of mindset were consistently helpful.

I'll never forget the advice I received from a doctor who had trained as a psychotherapist when I reported difficulties taking L-dopa, my primary medication. Granted, the medication had restored my mobility but at the cost of aggravating my panic and anxiety attacks which were already part of the underlying disease itself. He simply advised me to conclude a peace treaty or a pact with the few medications that could actually help me. And yes, there was something unscientific about his advising me to enlist L-dopa as an ally, but compared with the sterile logic of mainstream medical statistics it seemed like an attempt to retain some of the wisdom seen in magical practices. A magical approach to the world is one that refuses to accept the separation of subject and object that is widespread in modern times. Scientifically oriented human medicine is based on the acceptance of mute natural laws that apply without respect of person. According to this theory of science, a doctor's actions are similar to those of an engineer. Doctors do not view the body within its organic context, but see it as an isolated entity. In fact, the practice of medicine consists of a silent intervention in an array of objects, of things. The fact that human beings are endowed with intellect isn't a consideration in this approach. Enlightened physicians have long been aware that ignorance of this dimension can itself lead to disease. An alternative perspective could arise from the subjectivism of a worldview one can term "magical" in memory of an archaic, pre-Christian way of relating to the world. It is certainly no coincidence that calls for a different kind of medical epistemology are being raised in the disciplines that address diseases occurring at the very interface of body and soul, which is to say, psychiatry and neurology.

3.

I often find myself thinking what a vast number of coincidences determine our lives. I'm referring not only to
the chromosome lottery at the beginning of life, but
rather to the situation where, at the threshold of old age,
one asks: which aspects of my biography may be attributed
to my own merit or guilt, and which have resulted from
pure coincidence, like the hurricane in North America
that is caused by the stroke of a butterfly's wings on the
Island of Celebes—via an infinite chain of causation. This
image from the field of chaos research does not advocate
the self-empowerment of science, which supposedly has
everything under control. On the contrary! It posits that
the complexity of the insights we reconstruct always lags
far behind the complexity of the actual reconstructed
events themselves. Seen from this modest perspective,
everything becomes a coincidence.

This chaos-theory-based apologia for randomness is the
secret accomplice of a science that refuses to focus its
attention on the darker sides of life. Isn't every decision-
competent individual a co-author of coincidence, thereby
removing the coincidental element from coincidence? Don't
vitality and creativity consist of the strength and presence of
mind to utilize coincidences as opportunities, thereby dimin-
ishing coincidence to the mere fabric of one's own will?

On the other hand, personal experiences as well as professional reflection on life draw our attention to the vast degree our that everyday activities are determined by external and internal factors which lie beyond our reach. People simply like to forget that each individual action represents an unintentional, secondary consequence of previous actions—their own as well as those of others. They forget about the contingent surrounding circumstances. They tend to deny to themselves the great degree that decisions seemingly reached on one's own are or were in reality the product of subtle negotiation processes.

When we examine coincidence, we can't limit ourselves to factors that have exerted a positive influence on our lives. It was also a coincidence that I contracted a disease, and statistics is the art of expressing the degree of such coincidence. In my age group I was one out of approximately eight hundred. At a gathering of roughly eight hundred people, say, in a schoolyard, I was the sole individual to be singled out; with no explanation, no consolation, and no help whatsoever in making sense of it.

For as long as it is not determined that environmental toxins or other external factors are responsible for causing Parkinson's disease, and that I (knowingly) exposed myself to such factors through negligence and thoughtlessness, I remain simply the victim of coincidence and bear no responsibility. The turbulent growth of scientific knowledge about the human body has led to an explosive increase in the range of physical defects for which we are held accountable. The field of preventive health care offers perhaps the clearest case in point. The scientifically proven causal relationship between smoking and serious health damage has entirely eliminated any notion of chance from respiratory and cardiovascular disease. A bronchial carcinoma no longer "just happens" to someone. The people themselves are to blame; they themselves bear the responsibility. This inclination to banish coincidence from our interpretations of day-to-day events has long been part of our lives. When we encounter a friend who has fallen seriously ill, we all recognize in ourselves a tendency to secretly hold the friend him or herself accountable for the illness. Wasn't he a smoker, didn't he have a hectic lifestyle? We will accept the most absurd constructs in order to normalize our fear of a negative coincidence. Further examples can be seen in the fields of retirement planning and social policy. The most interesting documentation stems from the field of prenatal diagnostics. Recently developed tests make it possible to predict myriad types of damage to the fetus that will result in disease, allergic intolerance, or disabilities. Parents who ignore this assume grave responsibility.

We are standing on the threshold of a worrisome age.

In contrast to earlier times, contingency, that which is unexpected and new, is constantly increasing. The traditions that the past once used to bind the future to itself are disintegrating. Uncertainty has become the central concept of our hypermodern culture. Conventional theories would have us believe that we are merely in a transitional phase to new certainties. From the beginning of written history there have been epochs of collective existential insecurity, when traditional patterns of interpretation weakened before new certainties established themselves. Yet the special feature of our age seems to be that the hiatus between "no longer" and "not yet" is becoming a permanent condition.

Today, many of the new developments in economic and social policy, as well as in medicine, are having a combined effect in the sense that the burden of processing problems resulting from the invalidation of randomness must be borne by the individual. Responsibility is in short supply; it can't be imposed upon one person without having been lifted from someone else. The obverse of the paradoxical simultaneity of uncertainty on one side and dramatized responsibility on the other can be seen in a new irresponsibility. This has found its way over recent decades into entities such as government and health-care systems in all hypermodern societies.

4.

I don't like to see photos of myself, with rare exceptions. One such photo shows me renovating a cottage in Lower Bavaria that I rented with friends in the early '70s. I'm in my early thirties and "built," that is, athletic and on the heavy side. I'm taking a break, leaning against a wall and smoking a cigarette, while coolly and confidently observing the woman taking the picture. That's the way I'd like to see myself: virile and in full control of my life, a man who lifts his eyes to the stars but has both feet on the ground.

If I could live my life over again, or could order time to linger, then this is the age I'd chose. With the exception of my childhood, this was the only period of my life where I lived in peace with my body. A serious bout of acne had just cleared up thanks to new medication, and Parkinson's would still grant me a good decade of forbearance. During these years my body was a resource to be mined, a power supply you only notice when you push it to the limit.

The first and simultaneously most lasting feeling that the diagnosis of Parkinson's triggered was a sense of narcissistic injury, one that no other injury inflicted by a human being has ever surpassed. At a single blow, I felt excluded from the fellowship of those who simply had their bodies at their disposal, who experienced no friction losses between an impulse to act and the action itself. At first it was rare, but as the illness progressed my body proved itself increasingly often, although never predictably, to be a subject that was separate from me and walked its own inscrutable paths. Prior to major social or physical undertakings such as a party or a walk, I first had to test my body's willingness to perform.

In the past, I often made fun of women who can't pass a mirror without casting a self-satisfied, scrutinizing glance at themselves. Now it was I myself who couldn't pass a mirror. Although in my case it wasn't vanity that prevented me from passing one by, but rather a well-justified fear of my motor coordination and facial expression, which no longer complied with my conscious will and had gradually begun to lead lives of their own. In the few photos that were taken of me during the first years of my illness, I notice a mask-like rigidity, while in contrast I find my eyes to be larger, sadder, and more expressive than before I fell ill. At the time, I was deeply shocked by video recordings. For the first time I saw my grotesque dyskinesias.

My body has always been a sounding board for my erotic pleasure, which it incidentally continued to be during the dark years following the diagnosis. Erotic touching and encounters grew all the more important the thicker the glass wall became between me and my social environment.

To be viewed with love, or even erotic desire, is an important source of self-experience. In Renaissance painting there are depictions of noblewomen exhibiting themselves to a male slave after bathing or while dressing. By displaying themselves before a slave they demonstrated that they didn't view him as a human being. He simply did not belong to the circle of erotic combatants. Overcoming shame is a precondition for erotic love. The biblical phrase "to know a woman" refers to nothing other than this. I am the delight in the eye of the other. I experience myself as a person only indirectly, that is, as mediated by someone else who looks at me with love and whose eyes reflect me.

The joy of experiencing oneself through the loving attention of others is not, as is often suggested, the privilege of the rich, young, and beautiful. There are no Untouchables in our culture. There is no defect, no stigma, no personal disfigurement that can not be bridged by gestures of friendship and love.

5.

I often think of the song by Eric Burdon: "I was so much older then, when I was young." I think that the clock of a successful life displays two different times: one displays our inescapable biological decline, the other is the discovery of our own identity which proceeds in a counterclockwise direction. People who resist the temptation to remain the way they are can have crazy experiences: inhibitions are shed, blinders fall way, things that were once important become insignificant, what was once unimportant moves center stage. But such lightness doesn't simply fall into our laps. Over the course of their lives, sad people must experience so much external misfortune that the sum of that misfortune equals the amount of unhappiness they have always carried with them internally. Only then will the membrane that prevents a sad person from participating fully in life rupture, thereby liberating the happiness that will compensate him for his previous history of suffering.

The split I mentioned between the world and the self applies not only to my state of separateness from my fellow human beings, but also to their alienation toward me.

Ever since it has become impossible to conceal my condition from the world, it has triggered bizarre reactions in many people. Looking back on more than a decade of experience with Parkinson's, I would say that the transformation of one's social environment is more pointed and hurtful than all of the physical symptoms. It is even less than a truism to say that times of crisis separate the wheat from the chaff, which is to say that true friendships and relationships only prove their worth in the hour of need. The situation is obviously more complicated. Often it is the truly important ties, relationships, and social arrangements that do not stand the test of a bitter reality. And, correspondingly, those who remain loyal to us through thick and thin are often not the people whose presence, warmth, and solidarity we enjoy over the long term.

It is impossible to make general statements about how people will react to the fact that I suffer from Parkinson's disease. It depends on whether they are men or women, relatives, close friends, acquaintances, colleagues, or one's own children or parents. Even before that, there is the question of who is entitled to pass judgment as to whether the reactions are "good," "appropriate," or "bad." Another key factor is the circumstances prevailing at the time others take note of my illness. Is the information completely new to them? Did I already have the illness when we met, or did it erupt into a life we shared, just as startlingly and shockingly as it did for me?

One surprising experience in my case was that it tended to be men whose reactions I found tactful and appropriate, and whose gestures of solidarity I was able to accept without fear or ambivalence.

In moral philosophy one differentiates between two basic attitudes that people assume toward their own kind: that of caring and that of detachment. The relationship of this differentiation to that of "masculine" and "feminine" is not coincidental. In our culture, caring as well as detachment represent behavioral qualities that are demanded of women and men respectively in bringing up their children. Now, that doesn't mean that all men are incapable of developing virtues that stem from caring for friends, wards, children, etc. Correspondingly, there are definitely women who exhibit typically male character traits such as formal rationality or a predilection for power and competition. The attribution of female traits to women has nothing to do with their nature as determined by their biological gender. This widespread connection merely reflects the role women play within the structure of our gender-specific division of labor. We encounter the traits considered "typically female" in this complicated sense not only in behavior toward children, but also toward partners—and the sick.

With male friends I consistently experienced that they did not deny the existential divide that had opened between us based on my illness. Apparently, the inclination toward caring and empathy which is attributed to the female gender is not a good foundation for a long term relationship between male friends. That may be different in the field of professional care. In a number of cases, I observed that during periods of extreme pressure, behavior patterns based on the promise of a symbiotic willingness to provide care can lead to hypocrisy and result in a painful termination of the friendship. When I encountered male friends for the first time after they learned of my illness, they showed no reluctance to inquire about my motor symptoms with a kind of unconcealed clinical interest, to tactfully ask me for information, and to advise me to adopt a rational, wait-and-see attitude. A rational approach consisted initially of staying calm so that I could achieve two complementary objectives. First of all, to soberly gather clear information about the limitations I would have to expect, and then to sort them into those I would have to learn to bear, and those that could be changed. I was easily able to cope with that. But I was extremely sensitive to people's inability to respect boundaries, their presumption of symbiotic intimacy, and their false gestures of solidarity.

In general, however, the reactions of friends and acquaintances tended to be unpleasant in the opposite sense.

A large number of (not so close) friends and acquaintances reacted by gradually putting our contacts on ice. There are many potential interpretations of such behavior. Most likely it was a reflection of my own inability to come to terms with the illness. I have the impression that the underlying reason for this reaction pattern was because they didn't perceive the news of my illness as what it was, i.e., a misfortune that affected me alone, but rather as a statistical possibility that they themselves might fall victim to a similar stroke of fate.

The reaction of one's own children, one's own parents, and one's partner is a difficult chapter. My son's reaction as a child was relatively easy to work out. Children have an inclination toward an egocentrism all their own, which renders their attitudes, opinions, and mindsets predictable to a large extent. Once I had plausibly assured him that I wouldn't die of Parkinson's but simply become stiffer and jerkier, he was relieved. With the pragmatic eagerness of a child that perceives all existential threats exclusively from the perspective of his or her respective developmental level, he remarked, "Well, then that's not so bad at all." But later on, as he grew up, it did turn out to be bad. When he entered puberty, there was no over-looking the fact that some of my bizarre symptoms were embarrassing to him in public. He was also annoyed by my mumbling, which was often difficult to understand, and he found my tendency to withdraw from the world decidedly threatening.

The question of the ability of partnerships to endure stress does not require lengthy consideration. In some rela-tionships, news of this kind can be beneficial and lead to clarifications that the partners might otherwise not have had the strength to achieve. Time and again the platitude proves true that partnerships either stand up under such endurance tests and as a result tend to become stronger than before, or they collapse under the existential burden of this kind of diagnosis. There is no third option. And no one should shed tears for such relationships after the fact, least of all the victims of the disease themselves. Over the course of many therapeutic stays in Parkinson's clinics, I've had the opportunity to view the wreckage of collapsed rela-tionships. Mostly it involved women whose incorrect understanding of dedication had resulted in their forfeiting the opportunity to lead autonomous lives, while being unable to help their sick partners in any way. I experienced couples who, in their mute embitterment over their false lives, battered each other at night so severely that they were unable to appear for breakfast the next morning. Under-standing the limits of solidarity on the part of one's partner and immediate family is the central accomplishment demanded of the victims of illness, who prefer, despite all impairment, to spend their lives in a natural partnership.

I don't know which to admire more, the fortitude of the chronically ill who face their difficult lives alone, or the patience, love and solidarity that are required to lead such a life together. I believe that a couple's decision to separate when faced with the illness of one party does not warrant criticism. Nothing is worse, even for the party who is ill, than for the separation to be repeatedly deferred or not take place at all for sentimental reasons. I am indebted to my then girlfriend from Vienna for this experience. On the day I received my diagnosis, I called her and gave her the bad news. After a week of painful silence she called me back and put it very simply. She didn't want to dupe me. She didn't believe that her love was great enough to live with me "under these circumstances."

My attachment to my father had already begun to unravel while he was still alive. Due to his Alzheimer's he was already dead, in the sense of no longer being a capable person, before he actually passed away. I learned that I had Parkinson's ten years before his death. Ruth, the woman he married after my mother's early death, initially wanted to spare my father the bad news because he was already extremely frail and debilitated. At the time, I found that decision to be most welcome.

One day, however, Ruth called me outside of our normal calling routine and told me it was time to tell him the truth. I drove to see him that weekend and talked emphatically with him until Ruth urged me to stop. She had the impression that he was tired, sad, and confused. He had stopped listening to me a long time ago. Even though I was aware of his inclination to sidestep unpleasant news, the exacerbation of this tendency only became clear to me in the context of my illness. A peculiar transformation of our relationship set in from this point on. Every telephone conversation between us began with a dramatically phrased, "Well, how are you?"

He almost never waited for me to answer, as if he were afraid that I would burden him with bad news. During his seven remaining years, we exchanged not a single word about my illness. He simply didn't want to know. I'll never forget the last time I saw him. He was waiting for me—as in the past—at the garden gate, wearing felt slippers and resting his forearms on the fence. It was the end of February. The remains of the last snowfall were still all over the garden. A somewhat mild breeze, an early harbinger of an as yet distant spring, ruffled his thin hair. He looked at me. His eyes were empty. He didn't recognize me. The reflection in the eye of the other had been cut off for ever. He was disconcerted as he looked at me and said with great formality, "What can I do for you, Sir?"

One reaction I enjoy remembering was that of an elegant old woman who sat across the table from me in the dining car on a train to Munich. She asked whether she might join me. All of the other seats were taken. At first, we studied each other without saying anything. Then her eyes shifted to the landscape rushing by. Suddenly she spoke. She apologized for addressing me so personally, but she felt the need for conversation. She thought it was a fortunate coincidence that the only vacant seat in the entire dining car was at my table. I impressed her as someone she could talk to. She said she wasn't well versed in the art of casual chitchat. If I objected, she would return to her compartment and come back when there was room at another table. I'd been caught slightly off guard, but my curiosity got the better of me. And then she told me a sad story. She was coming from the university clinic in Würzburg where she had just learned that her daughter was suffering from cancer and didn't have long to live. Her daughter had asked her to break the news to her grandchildren, both of whom were still very young. And that now lay before her. Although she related this with great internal turmoil, she remained composed and shed no tears. In this way she prepared the ground for me to relate my own sad little story, in a similarly distanced and discreet manner. The tone she had adopted helped me speak about my illness in a way that I experienced the accumulated sadness of my story, while at the same time the weight of the world was lessened in the telling. When we parted on the platform in Munich, I would have liked to embrace her. I didn't have the courage.

In this little episode it is easy to identify the conditions that made our communication successful. First, it was the anonymity of our encounter. Granted, we had introduced ourselves, although I didn't catch her name at the beginning and I'm sure she didn't catch mine, either. And then, our situation was symmetrical. She had worries and wanted to discuss them; I was in a similar situation. We had met by chance, and our acquaintance also came to an end after less than two hours. This allowed us to take turns and calmly unpack our worries, so to speak, and yet with empathy, without the least prospect of having to assume responsibility for one another afterwards. It was and remained an encounter between strangers. And as a result, it couldn't actually be taken as a model for interactions in daily life. The situation would be different if the encounter were interpreted as one between friends. In that case, the very characteristics displayed in the meeting, such as empathy and concurrent distance, would stand as the conditions of successful interaction between humans, who as such are also always suffering beings.

6

According to the statistics, Parkinson's only strikes when you have descended from the high plateau of life, when the children are out of the house, and you've begun thinking about retirement anyway. Parkinson's is known as a neurodegenerative disease of old age.

I, however, was struck in the midst of life. I had just been appointed a full professor, while retaining my position as deputy director of a small but prestigious research institute. At the time, my ambition and energy level were ample for two jobs. I was successful. I was publishing books and monographs on a regular basis, and they found readers. The executive director was already far beyond retirement age. This age constellation in itself confirmed the generally held opinion that I was the crown prince of the institute.

Once I received the diagnosis, however, a gradual process of alienation arose between the institute and me, which would conclude three years later with a humiliating dismissal.

During the year following the diagnosis I changed radically. It was surely not a transformation caused by verifiable changes in brain physiology, but rather a psychological adjustment to a biorhythm that had become utterly unpredictable due to the illness and medication. I could no longer predict whether I'd be in sufficiently good shape—in the next few minutes, in the next hour, or in the afternoon—to receive guests, lead a discussion, or chair a meeting. I would soon learn that there is a technical term for the specific kind of "bad shape" Parkinson's sufferers find themselves in; it's called an "off phase." And indeed, it feels as if someone had pulled the plug on your body's mental apparatus and it's only running on "stand-by," on back-up current, so to speak. All movements become toilsome, your face freezes, it becomes difficult to speak, even intellectual processes decelerate. When that happens, the only thing that helps is an L-dopa preparation, although it takes an hour for the effect to set in. There is still nothing to counteract the engulfing social embarrassment in the presence of people who haven't the slightest idea of what you are experiencing at that moment. With time, every victim of the disease develops strategies to cope with this ordeal. Most people decide in favor of complete withdrawal from the world. Mostly, I made an intuitive decision to do opposite, or at least I tried. Even when I found myself in an "off phase," I would nevertheless muster my remaining energy to explore my inner world, to experience the way my inner condition at that moment would overwhelm me to such a degree that stimuli and reactions from the external world would seem secondary. My innermost perceptions, my experience of myself, my solipsism commanded absolute primacy.

The little parties where people at the institute stood around and celebrated important events became hellish for me after the onset of Parkinson's. The diffuse array of people in the room, their erratic movements, my increasingly unsuccessful efforts to coordinate my facial expression, physical movements, and speech left me petrified with fear. I had to keep the fear itself under control. It was so completely inappropriate in a setting of superficial, compulsory good humor. The most awful part of it was the expectation that I would ad-lib a short speech. That had been a specialty of mine during the years before. Now I would prepare for days, and only simulate the spontaneity of the presentation. The illness forced me to budget my energy. At these gatherings, where we remained standing, I wasted the better part of my mental and intellectual energies simply on not constantly bumping into other people in the room and controlling my facial expression and enunciation. If the parties lasted for a while, I began having extremely regressive wishes, for example, to cry, scream or simply lie down right in the middle of everyone and go to sleep. It would have been helpful in those situations, if I could have discussed my mental state with people I trusted. It was only years later that I was able to do so.

In keeping with my social status and based on my professional activities as a researcher, teacher, and a manager within the framework of two positions, I was in the midst of life. But I was increasingly excluded from it by virtue of my inner condition. The bulk of my energy was consumed by concealing this dichotomy. I became estranged from many colleagues and friends whom I had known for ages. I often listened to their conversations in amazement. I was stunned by how much of their lives, how much speaking time, they devoted to matters I considered absolutely trivial. Professorial colleagues in my immediate surroundings warranted especially little mercy in my eyes. I found their vanity and their hauteur unbearable. Had I once been that way myself?

Two things changed fundamentally. My superficial cheerfulness, which had repeatedly needed recharging through minor academic successes, had now been replaced in my inner household by an existential gravity for which I had made no provisions. This was augmented by a feeling of not having much time left. It was plain to me that I would not lead the institute into the new millennium, even though I generally suppressed this knowledge. In the morning, I still had a real thirst for action and strode vigorously into the small, inconspicuous building. But by the early afternoon my hands already began to shake so severely that even typing on a keyboard became exhausting. Although this alienation from my world became more exacerbated by the day, it was not only a disadvantage. It secured things for me that would not have been available in the absence of my existential burden, namely, independence of judgment as well as intellectual sovereignty and incorruptibility.

At that time, I began to write papers that were sharply critical of current conditions at the institute. The first people to read these papers were colleagues, generally erstwhile friends, who were deeply shocked by the unmerciful tenor of my argumentation and the uncompromising position I took. A strange antagonistic constellation arose: in the name of goals that needed to be achieved in the future, the management of the institute opposed the employees, who had closed ranks and were struggling to retain the old structures.

The countless debates conducted in those days number among the worst experiences of my career. The arguments we exchanged had been known for a long time. One position faced off against the other. I find academic discourse tolerable only to the extent that it does not exclude the possibility of learning from one's opponent, so that one can exit the rhetorical battlefield a different person, one who has been taught something, with head held high. The grave controversy in the small institute with the big name, which soon led to repercussions in the university as well, had no such spirit. Arguments were weapons meant to intimidate the opponent. The greatest recognition one could expect from an adversary was an acquittal based on lack of evidence. But the problem wasn't caused exclusively by other people. My own obstinacy, born of loneliness, also contributed to the atmosphere. Perhaps I was even the primary cause. In those days we were hosting an American guest scholar who was thoroughly shaken by the aggressive impasse the controversy had reached. Given the rigid, immobile fronts, and faced with the mute tenacity of both camps, he was reminded of a human body that contracts all of its muscles at the same time and thereby paralyzes itself. "It's like Parkinson's disease. Your institute is sick. It's crippled by Parkinson's."

He knew nothing of my diagnosis.

In the mid-90s the situation unexpectedly came to a head, and a decision followed. On a cool spring day, I received a call from the then president of the university, whom I knew in passing. He invited me to dine with him, along with the minister of culture, a representative of the minister president, and the city's representative for cultural affairs.

During the meal, regret was expressed over the decline of the institute's great tradition, and a general desire was affirmed that a new beginning should be undertaken. My suggestions were received with polite reserve. I quickly understood that the decision to unseat my colleague as director had already been made and that the throne was vacant, so to speak. For the first time during the bitter struggle over the future of the institute, I was in a position where all I had to do was to help myself to the power that lay before me.

The only thing this illustrious circle expected of me was that I seize the opportunity. The fact that I didn't seize it determined the outcome of the whole story. For the first time, I openly exhibited my existential insecurity, without naming its cause. It would have been then, at the latest, that perceptive observers could have recognized the cleft between me and the world, which I was still hiding with all my might, even when I would have been at liberty to divulge it. But I did not possess that stature.

One of the more recent presidents of Harvard University succumbed to a major depression during his tenure, which severely interfered with the otherwise flawless discharge of his duties. He thereupon petitioned the trustees for a one-year leave of absence. His request was granted and, in the solitude of a country estate and a Buddhist monastery, he managed to recover so that he could serve out his term. By the way, all phases of this process played out in full public view. I wish I could have been as self-confident as the president of that university.

Afterwards, the situation cooled down somewhat. The open civil war in the little institute with the grand tradition scaled back to a kind of twilight war, waged from that point onward in taverns and around communal dinner tables. I shifted to my fallback position, namely, teaching courses, and went to the institute only when necessary.

I was tired and burned out. Conflicts are not my thing, and a war on two fronts even less so. For I was not only in conflict with my colleagues, but also with myself, over the best way to withdraw from the battlefield without too great a loss of face. More than once, as I made the trip from the train station to my apartment, I fantasized arriving and finding out that the institute had burned to the ground. Apparently, my fantasy reflected a wish. The destroyed institute of my daydream would have relieved me of making a decision in one direction or the other. I could either make public reference to my illness and resign from the institute, or continue to wage a conflict that I alone recognized as long lost, because the overwhelming adversary had entrenched itself in my own mind.

From that point on, I cannot discern any plan or rationality in my actions. I no longer recognize myself as an accountable, plan-making subject. I reeled from situation to situation like a punch-drunk boxer, telling one person this, and the next person that, depending on my overall mood which was constantly changing. Occasionally, I even breached the hermetic discretion about my illness, with the selection of those in whom I confided just as random as the information I revealed.

During that period I accepted a six-month guest professorship at the University of California, Berkeley—against the advice of many well-meaning friends. They spoke of numerous intrigues, all of which were directed at undermining the strong position I still held, as seen from the outside. They said it was a tactical error to leave the country under this particular set of circumstances. Based on my knowledge of my true condition, I felt invulnerable from without. No hostility could compete with the aggression I directed toward myself. I would either be strong enough to hand in my resignation on my own, based on my illness, or I would simply be thrown out because a relevant majority no longer wanted me. What elese could happen to me?

The decision came quickly. And I myself did much to ensure that it was a depressing and humiliating departure. In September of that year, a birthday and an anniversary happened to coincide: both the previous director and the institute itself turned seventy-five. An informal gathering alone would not suffice to mark the occasion. A major, public conference would show due respect for the double anniversary. The conference was to be held six weeks after my departure. Naturally, I was willing to interrupt my stay at Berkeley specifically for this purpose. I had been assigned a major address at the convention and had selected a topic that I'd never worked on before.

At Berkeley a leaden serenity came over me. For a significant part of the day, I would lie in the shadow of a magnolia tree and watch the raccoons cavorting on the roof of the house. The hummingbirds, likewise, hovering before open blossoms like bumblebees, were also more interesting in every respect than the stack of books I had demonstratively piled beside my deck chair. When the display on my phone indicated that someone from Frankfurt was calling, I didn't pick up the receiver. But the composure, which I interpreted as the final form of happiness still attainable for me, did not come from within. Unbeknownst to me as yet, it was the effect of a strong sedative that a pharmacist had given me in copious supply to take along on my trip. The effect of bromazepam is fantastic. One tablet bestows a good night's sleep, nightmare-free, and then even a carefree morning to follow.

I'm a professional. I realize that it is better to prepare thoroughly for reports at academic conferences that will be attended by colleagues or journalists who are in attack mode. During a phase where the effect of the bromazepam had worn off—it was around noon, and I was talking with a colleague in an outdoor restaurant on campus—I realized with the utmost clarity that for the audience in Frankfurt my lecture would unavoidably be a lecture cum job application.

When I boarded the flight in Oakland that would take me to Frankfurt, I hadn't yet written a single line. Only in the unreal atmosphere of the plane's fuselage, as it droned through the night, did I coax a couple of lines out of my laptop. In order to catch a few hours of sleep in spite of flying all night, I took two happy pills together. I experienced the darkest day of my career with such equanimity—as if the hummingbirds and the raccoons had taken me into their midst. During the lecture, I made every mistake a person can possibly make. Not only did I have no proposition or point one would have been able to discuss, but I spoke for forty minutes instead of twenty, which was the limit. How much I would have spared myself if I had only had the courage beforehand to say that I was sick and was resigning from the institute! In an indirect way I accomplished that through my lecture: I remained sitting when I was called to step up onto the podium; I mumbled under my breath and trembled visibly. An occasional boo was heard. During the discussion, one of my colleagues said that I was unworthy of presiding over the institute as its director. No one spoke out in my defense, except a colleague, a one-time friend, who said, to sparse applause, that we all have our bad days now and then and that he wanted to hark back to the papers from which many of those in the auditorium had profited. It was like an epitaph. After the brief discussion concluded, a cluster of faces approached me, acquaintances and strangers, all wanting to know what the matter was, and whether I was perhaps sick.

That evening there was another of those receptions where everyone stands around. Thanks to a third bromazepam I passed the evening in a state of great serenity, somewhat happily, almost. It felt like a Halloween party, and I was the only person invited who wasn't in costume. All the other party guests had long thin legs and disproportionately large pumpkin heads. The few people who exchanged more than greetings with me often brought their big pumpkin heads too close, so that I became frightened. The day before, I had still been one of them. Now I no longer belonged. Judging by my inner feelings, it had already been a long time since I'd been one of them.

I left the university guest house around midnight. The air was crisp, there was already a hint of autumn. My mind was clear, and I wasn't dizzy. It was almost a little bit like being well again, and I felt like going for a run. I went to my hotel, picked up my baggage, and booked an earlier flight. I slept the whole trip back to Oakland.

This short phase of defiant euphoria was followed by a lengthy depression after my return to Berkeley. I learned only gradually how to place the disgraceful and humiliating end of my public life in Frankfurt in a causal relationship to my illness. Instead of accepting this insight, I cultivated a melancholy machismo whereby it is only the existential setbacks that make a man a man; "becoming a man means learning how to lose." But it was obvious that this existential kitsch was only a further attempt to evade the full impact of the truth.

The full impact of the truth would have consisted of realizing that an extremely limiting and incurable disease such as Parkinson's, when it is full-blown, robs a person of the ability to continually reinvent himself. It forces him into a cramped cycle of ever-identical activities, whose only logic consists of offering the least amount of resistance to a physical body that has been rendered unreliable. One's life becomes similar to that of a plant: silent, without transcendence and autonomy. In a sense, it's not even a life anymore—just existence in an atrophied form. Yet in my case that truth did not apply.

7

Thanks to a fortunate coincidence, I was spared returning to Frankfurt for the time being. A colleague drew my attention to an announcement of a two-year guest professorship at New York University, which would follow my stay in California almost seamlessly. My application, compiled with minimal emotional investment, was successful. Despite the constant presence of Parkinson's symptoms, the years I subsequently spent in New York number among the most beautiful and successful of my entire career.

Now that I am able to look back on several years of experience with the disease, I am forced to admit to myself that I had been fortunate things hadn't turned out worse. My Parkinson's was progressing at a slower rate than the original prognoses had led me to expect. New drugs certainly played a role as well. My brain was the scene of a peculiar race: the gradual degeneration of the substantia nigra competing against the effectiveness of new pharmaceuticals and the speed at which they were being released. Additionally, during the years in New York I was socially well integrated and well under control with my medications.

In New York everybody's a little crazy. My tremor and fidgety, restless limbs hardly raised an eyebrow. The different mode of dealing with disease and disablement in public also helped me to develop a different attitude toward Parkinson's.

I see three stages in my relationship to Parkinson's up to that point. The first consisted of complete ignorance of all indications of the disease, even though they were physically palpable. Symptomatic for this was my denial of being sick when confronted with the diagnosis by the doctor in Frankfurt. I roundly disputed having the disease even though I had read with my own eyes the day before in a bookstore in Vienna that the very symptoms I was exhibiting suggested a diagnosis of Parkinson's. Once the presence of Parkinson's had been confirmed by a professional, I could no longer maintain the strategy of denial I had pursued until then. Nevertheless, the second stage of my relationship with Parkinson's did not consist of unqualified acceptance. As far as I could, I kept my diagnosis secret in public. It was a schizoid attitude: a (still partial) admission of the disease to myself and those who were close to me, with denial and secrecy toward my social environment. Although this allowed me to carry on with my established career for the time being, it naturally entailed the painful cost of splitting my self.

Fragmenting my self, to put it more aptly. Because in Frankfurt, circles of colleagues overlap more so than they do elsewhere. What would have been an intelligent information policy with regard to my condition? I recall a minor scandal at an institute in Munich where I worked years ago. A professor who was somewhat older and a staunch Catholic fell in love with a young female student. He divorced his wife—Pope or no Pope—and married the young woman. In order to contain the gossip he anticipated, he did something very clever. He took the young woman by the hand, went from office to office with her, and introduced her to each of his coworkers. I don't recall that this colleague and his young wife continued to be the object of any further public attention.

If I had only had the self-assurance during one of those standing receptions at the institute in Frankfurt back then to declare without reserve what was the matter with me and that I was resigning!

It was only under the special circumstances I encountered in New York that I was able to avoid this fragmentation of my self from the outset. And yet in light of my illness, I was uncertain whether to accept the offer to go to New York at all. I cast the warnings of well-intentioned friends and my own trepid ego to the wind. Giving good advice to those who are ill, particularly when the diagnosis is so dramatic, is no less difficult than it is for the victim of the illness to accept the advice. Since it is impossible to arrive at an absolutely objective picture of a person's actual state, either through self-assessment or an assessment by others, every evaluation is of necessity a balancing act between dramatization and trivialization. Dramatization and trivialization, as the unavoidable outcomes when the evaluation of a prevailing condition misses the mark, are additionally also psychologically motivated. For obvious reasons, those who are ill prefer the trivializing option because it strengthens their illusion that things aren't that bad after all. Meanwhile, what sick people can't accept is that trivialization leads to the expectation that they will shoulder inappropriate burdens. Dramatization, on the other hand, no matter how philanthropically motivated it might be, necessarily leads to a symbolic disenfranchisement of the person who is ill. The tableau of motives would become even more complicated if one were to examine the average motivations of helpers and advisors. Thus, trivialization spares helpers from having to confront the full impact of the drama that has engulfed a fellow human being. Amazingly, dramatization can have a similar effect. By emphasizing that the sick person is different, that is, by underscoring his otherness, helpers can eschew the possibility of realizing the fragility of human existence, which the sick do indeed embody, but also share in common with healthy people.

The only advice I could accept without reservation came from a female colleague in Berkeley who was ill herself, suffering from advanced multiple sclerosis. She recommended that I take the position in any case, but that I be candid with all of the offices and people in charge, even if it entailed the danger that they would decide against me at the last second. And that's exactly what I did. Months before I was to take the post, I traveled to New York and spoke to the department head, several of my future colleagues, and the dean, mentioning my problem. The uniformly friendly reactions I experienced, in addition to the willing offers to provide active assistance, carried all the more weight for me since they were based on extensive knowledge of the symptoms and course of Parkinson's. Apart from that, they all made it unmistakably clear that they would expect the same output from me as any other healthy colleague. After the torturous years at the institute in Frankfurt, which had been torturous primarily because of my compulsive silence about my illness, the urbane, stimulating work atmosphere and the uninterrupted stream of recognition and encouragement in New York

made me feel as if I were in an oxygen tent that was help-
ing me to breathe again. I fulfilled the expectations that
had been placed on me. When my contract expired after
two years, it was renewed. I was the first person to hold
the guest professorship and have his contract extended
after the two-year term.

In major US cities one finds an exemplary public toler-
ance toward people with stigmas, handicaps, and disabilities. In Manhattan, for example, I had to take a bus every
morning during rush hour, always at the same time; as a
rule it was packed. And every morning the same scene
transpired. A severely disabled person would be waiting at
a bus stop in a wheelchair that he could only operate using
a small joystick. The bus driver had to get out of the bus
and move a lever that lowered a hydraulic platform and
allowed the wheelchair user to drive onto the bus. There,
the driver had to secure the wheelchair with belts, raise the
platform back up, and return to the steering wheel. The
whole procedure took about five minutes. I always had to
hold my breath when the wheelchair user got off at the
next stop, and the self-same procedure was repeated, only
in reverse. During my entire stay I never noticed a single
sign of impatience among fellow passengers.

It was in New York that I also experienced a collapse of
my entire motor apparatus, a total "off" condition, for the
first and, to date, only time. It happened on the way to the
movies. It was Saturday evening, a hot summer day in
Manhattan. Initially, my son was accompanying me. He
was visibly irritated by my slow, shuffling gait. For my
part, I was feeling rushed. In addition, I was bothered by
the many pedestrians who were coming toward us, con-

stantly requiring me to change direction. At Astor Place I became dizzy. I suggested to my son that he go ahead by himself and wait for me at the cinema on Broadway. He agreed. My vertigo increased and was accompanied by a new kind of difficulty coordinating my eyes. My pupils began contracting and dilating involuntarily and independently of one another. From one moment to the next, I was hardly capable of placing one foot in front of the other. It was as if I were wearing shoes of lead. A strong sensation of weakness in my legs forced me to scout for a safe haven, which turned out to be an unimposing complex of buildings I had passed scores of times on the bus, without ever consciously registering it.

It consisted of a small parking garage, repair shop, gas station, and kiosk in one. It was unusual in every respect, not least because of the multitude of functions its builders had intended for it. It was also surprising that international real-estate investors had overlooked the building complex. Groupings such as this are easy to find on the waterfront in Brooklyn, on the other side of the East River, but not here in southern Manhattan. And finally, it was out of the ordinary because the building, with its measly three stories, seemed to be cowering between the surrounding skyscrapers, as if it were trying from the outset to avoid any comparisons and any appearance of competing with them. These were all considerations and observations that I did not make with a lucid mind until my head had cleared and I was able to move again.

Panic-stricken, disoriented, and manifestly unable to stand on my legs any longer, I simply sat down on a vacant seat, fished my little pillbox out of my trouser pocket and immediately took a very big dose of L-dopa.

The colorful clutch of people who had already been sitting on the bench for a long time, silently registered my intrusion, which had clearly been an emergency measure. My trembling hands as I held my pillbox were commentary enough. Their questioning faces were not sufficiently urgent to break my silence.

In addition to that, their attention had been captured by a musician, an older, bald Chinese man at the other end of the long bench, who was already surrounded by a small group of pedestrians. He was playing an unfamiliar instrument that was a hybrid between a cello and a violin. He was extracting tones of such sadness and sweetness that passersby were enchanted and stopped. All across the world there are kinds of music that allow us to feel the weight of a pent-up sadness and liberate us for a moment.

My memory of that evening, which began with such difficulties and ended so well, will forever be connected with the music of that Chinese man.

From that day on, I often went to the unimposing garage on Saturday evenings. There was almost always a vacant seat for me on the black bench. The magic of this inconspicuous place, which I visited frequently during the following months, emerged particularly on summer nights when darkness only fell late. Just as moths and insects leave their daytime hiding places when dusk has turned irrevocably into night, so they gathered: the taxi drivers, the delivery boys, and kitchen hands from the fast food places nearby, young police cadets from the police academy near Gramercy Park, the brothers and boy-friends of the cashiers at the gas station, students from dormitories in the area, and sometimes even grave diggers from a small cemetery, although they had been off work since six o'clock. Even today, a feeling of happiness comes over me when I think of those people sitting on the black bench in the half darkness, listening to the music of the Chinese man as insects buzzed around the neon lights.

It is an uncontested finding in suicide research that suicide rates drop substantially during periods of war and catastrophe across all countries and all epochs. The documented experiences of therapists and psychiatric epidemiologists testify to a similar paradox. During hard times—hard in the sense that large parts of the population are suffering under generally deplorable living conditions—levels of suffering appear to decrease in people who had previously been suffering from their own individual afflictions. Why is that so? Why is it a source of comfort when personal misfortune is embedded within collective suffering?

Every hardship that an individual encounters, such as a serious chronic illness, an accident, a separation, etc., always affects the person in two respects: existentially and statistically. In actual experience, these two dimensions are generally not separated. My sorrow over my personal affliction and my rage that it struck precisely me rarely arise separately.

In my case, the experience that my own level of suffering would decrease lastingly when it was framed by the sudden violent occurrence of a collective catastrophe was provided by the events of September 11, 2001. Up until that point my diagnosis was particularly painful to me because it affected me as an individual. I suffered under the existential injustice that the world continued to turn and had left me behind. In the days following my diagnosis I often dreamed of falling off an ocean liner on the high seas at night. Burned into my memory is the dream image of the ocean liner full of happy, laughing people who are rapidly pulling away from me. True, the events of September 11 weren't able to make me whole, but they did reconnect the thread of my life with the tales of suffering of neighbors and acquaintances whose loved ones lay buried in the rubble.

I was returning from a small lecture in the history department at Columbia University. It had been a kind of home game. Half of the audience knew my theories from the literature, the other half was curious. I was satisfied, almost a little elated.

When one leaves the Columbia campus at 116th St., Broadway cuts a swath through the mountain range of buildings that falls off to the south. Within a short time, the dark blue morning sky had given way to a towering, Cyclops-like mass of clouds. I asked the subway station attendant, who was dozing in his glass cage in the breeze of a fan, whether a person could walk to the southern tip of Manhattan in two hours. At first, he gave me a bewildered look but then suggested that I take the train to Union Square, get off, and walk down the rest of Broadway from there—using the Twin Towers of the World Trade Center as a landmark.

When I re-emerged at Union Square, the enormous clouds were rimmed with yellow borders. It still hadn't started to rain. A strong, warm wind had come up and was blowing dust, plastic bags, and trash paper that hadn't been weighed down yet with rain. To avoid constantly colliding with other pedestrians who were trying to shield their eyes from the dust, I switched from a crowded

Broadway over to Fifth Avenue. Once I got to Washington Square, I planned to cross back over to Broadway again.

It was there that I witnessed a scene so bizarre and so far removed from everyday life that later, when I was waking up or dropping off to sleep, I was sometimes uncertain whether it hadn't been a dream. Washington Square is a large, park-like space arranged around a central fountain, with fenced playgrounds, dog parks, and benches for those strolling by. The entire square itself is surrounded by a fence. One can only enter at the corners and at the midpoint of each of the sides. In earlier times the Square didn't enjoy the best of reputations. Even today the groups of drug dealers were not to be overlooked. But they were held in check by a host of plainclothes police officers who made no secret of their identity, as well as by mounted police. A few of the officers had dismounted to shelter themselves from the dust in the lee of a horse trailer. They had loosely hitched their horses to a bench. The horses sensed the approaching storm and were restless. When the first lightning bolt struck, followed only after long seconds by muffled thunder, one of the horses, a gray one, reared, tore itself loose, and galloped riderless into the park with hanging reins. At first it limited itself to galloping around the fountain, as if it didn't yet trust its sudden freedom. The police were even more panic-stricken than the horse. At lightning speed, they occupied the exits and were shouting frantically in an attempt to keep the horse from breaking out into the city. The shouting and further lightning bolts increased the animal's panic. It jumped over the fence into the dog park, whose denizens pursued it yapping wildly. It then jumped back into the square and circled the fountain another several times. It was only when the rain began that the animal calmed down somewhat and fell into a nervous trot. A young man with long hair who was tattooed and naked to the waist ran along beside the horse, grasped its reins, and brought it back to the swearing policemen.

I had sought protection under a leafy sycamore tree, from the rain as well as the horse. I was aware of the danger involved in standing under a tree during a thunderstorm, and even though the intervals between lightning and thunder were still large, and there was no real danger, I left Washington Square and walked back to Broadway. In the meantime, the rain developed into a tropical downpour. The sewer drains at the curbs could no longer contain the masses of water. Small lakes formed around them which couldn't be avoided when one crossed the street. The warm rain was lashed by the wind and seemed as if it were coming in sideways, not from above. There was no sense in seeking shelter from the rain in doorways or building entrances. By now, the expensive jacket I was wearing was nothing but a wet rag that I carried scrunched up under my arm. My trousers had been transformed into shapeless tubes, making it difficult to walk. Broadway, full of pedestrians just a moment before, was now populated only by undaunted joggers. I passed countless street cafes where most of the pedestrians had fled. My desire to continue walking in the rain was stronger. I was reminded of my childhood when I had once completely ignored a summer rain and continued to walk, despite my new shoes and my Sunday best. The thrashing I received could never completely erase the high I experienced that day. My mother loved retelling the story of the ruined shoes over and over within the family circle, partially amused but partially still appalled. Whereas for her it had become a misdeed that fell under the statute of limitations and was therefore fit to be told, for me it represented a euphoric experience of autonomy, before I had the words to express it. Later, when I did have the words, the experience was buried to a large extent and only resurfaced after numerous therapy sessions. But now the memory of that rainy summer day forty years before drove me unrelentingly onward, past countless shops, restaurants, and cafes whose glass windows mirrored my image back to me, something akin to a scarecrow in a necktie. I passed the wet shiny trees in front of City Hall, passed the Woolworth Building with its spire hidden in the low hanging clouds. I was happy. I jumped from the edge of the curb into the street, on one leg each time, like a child. A passage came to mind that Jorge Luis Borges had written at age eighty-five: "If I could live my life again, I would try to make more mistakes. I would be a little crazier than I have been, I would take far fewer things seriously. If I could start again from the beginning, I would try to have only good moments. For that is what life consists of, moments only; don't forget the present one."

The subway station attendant in the glass enclosure at the 116th St./Columbia University stop had told me that to reach the vicinity of my hotel I should take a left when I reached the World Trade Center. But all I saw was a nonspecific conglomeration of high-rises that had all been reduced to the same height by the low cloud covering. The most important distinguishing feature of the Twin Towers, their height, was now obscured by the clouds. Mistrusting my own memory, I decided to go right at Old St. Patrick's Church. The neighborhood seemed familiar to me, and at the same time foreign. I had been there before, but the sun was shining then and the streets had bustled. The dusky storm clouds had quenched all the colors. The rain-soaked, empty streets and the high-rises cowering under the low sky looked as if they had been filmed with an old video camera. Those grainy black-and-white images are now often put to stylistic use in new films and reality TV. They are consistently used to indicate an immediately impending danger. I had lost my way. I was exhausted. There were several taxis parked in front of a massive complex of buildings. I asked for the World Trade Center. A Rastafarian with loud music booming from his cab laughed at me. "It's right here," he said, pointing to the building where we were standing. It was only by promising a lavish tip that I persuaded a different driver to take me to the apartment complex on Water Street where I lived. I really must have looked like a scarecrow. But I was happy. It was September 10, 2001.

After the attacks of September 11, the southern section of Manhattan was completely closed to traffic. Only rescue workers, the police, firemen, and the National Guard were allowed access to the immediate "war zone." The streets belonged to pedestrians, skaters, bicyclists, and wheel-chair users. In spite of the countless people strolling down Fifth Avenue in the direction of the mushroom cloud, by themselves, as couples, or in small groups, it was oppressively quiet. The only sounds were the murmuring of hushed voices, the distant wail of sirens, and the muffled noise of fighter planes flying high over head. The voices were no longer those of the initial commotion. They were not yet the voices of sorrow and despair. Many articulated a rather numbing sense of having witnessed a historical break, although no one knew what was coming to an end, not to mention what might lie ahead.

To happier generations, history may seem like a wide river, where the lives of individual people float languidly along, connected at their edges with the histories of others. Currently, the river is changing course, seeking a new bed in whirlpools and torrential cascades.

How is it possible that the strongest military power in the world—one that plans to invest inconceivable sums of money in a satellite-supported defense shield so that it can protect itself from so-called rogue states—is not even capable of protecting its own Department of Defense from hijackers armed only with carpet cutters?

The shattered towers of the World Trade Center provided insight into the anatomy of modern societies, and not only in an architectural sense. They revealed a—secret— characteristic of their social architecture. The World Trade Center embodied, as did only a few other buildings in the world, the claim to power asserted by a class of experts whose management knowledge holds our global society together at its core, so to speak. One central characteristic of global scientific-technological civilization is the historically unprecedented concentration of management knowledge in the hands of transnational elites. As a result of the development and global dissemination of communications, mass communications, and transportation technologies, enormous information gains have occurred. Measured in terms of this complexity, which is now surveyable only in a virtual sense, modern man's everyday orientation represents nothing short of archaic simplicity. Complementary to this explosion of potential knowledge, a no less dramatic constriction of reality is taking place within the sphere that

individuals can experience locally and palpably, and pro-
ductively control.

Ulrich Beck referred to societies of this type as "risk
societies." They do not bear this name because conducting
life in modern societies is riskier than in pre-modern ones
but because of the social form in which collective risks are
managed today. Experts receive a mandate after their qual-
ifications and ethical integrity have been professionally
certified. Drawing on a term from information technology,
such risk management elites are also referred to as "expert
systems." Human beings become systems because their
knowledge lays claim to validity, irrespective of the authority of the concrete individuals who are applying it. In the
meantime, such expert systems permeate all areas of our
lives: how and what we eat; the medications we take; our
educational practices; how we get around and what we use
to do so, etc. Doctors, psychotherapists, and advisers of all
kinds also belong here.

Through the events of September 11, 2001, many people suddenly realized at the beginning of the twenty-first
century that the performance of everyday activities (driving a car, availing oneself of complex medical services, and
consuming food, as well as flying in commercial aircrafts,
using elevators in high-rise buildings or bridges in earth-
quake zones) depend on an existential trust in the technical competence and moral integrity of those who have
been put in charge of these functions.

At the beginning of the twenty-first century, many people, including those who don't read philosophical books,
sense that modernity's promise of salvation warrants mis-
trust because modernity itself has been reduced to technological progress and economic growth. Even bio- and

nanotechnology will not banish the fear of death and compensate for lost meaning. And even if events such as September 11 do not recur, as the citizens of New York venture to their secure, air-conditioned, and fully computerized offices, their movements will be jittery and anxious for a long time to come, much like prehistoric humans in the thickets of the primordial world.

For the first time, it occurred to me that everything I myself had thought about the future of my Parkinson's had been wrong. Up until then, I had held a conviction seated deep within my brain that someday the chance of a cure would emerge and that a look back at, say, twenty years of illness would then seem like a nightmare, a nightmare with paradisiacal happiness waiting for me when it was over. It is true that boasting neurologists and stem cell researchers have created the erroneous impression that the path to a cure begins just beyond the next bend in the road. But the pressure of public expectations notwithstanding, such hopes have not been fulfilled.

Today I believe that hopes of a cure held by the neurologically ill were not only delusive but also unfulfillable in principle. It is naïve and even wrong to expect that the years that medical advances could grant us would, as a matter of course, be good and successful ones. Where does such certainty come from? Sometimes I'm afraid that I have lost my ability to be happy during the long years of illness and hopelessness. Modern medicine will not be able to assist our search for lost happiness.

8.

After three years I had to return to Germany. My
university would not have been willing to grant me
a third year of unpaid leave. Thus, in order to
ensure the continuation of my activities in New York I
would have had to resign my tenured professorship in
Germany, which would have represented the courage to
face life that Jorge Luis Borges demands. Yet it wasn't only
my need for existential security that made remaining in the
United States completely out of the question, but also my
father, whose life was obviously drawing to a close—as
well as my son, who would soon graduate from high
school.

Up until the operation, the question of retiring from my
profession had never arisen. Due to the time limitations on
my involvement in New York, which were stipulated by
the German civil-service contract, I had a relatively short
planning horizon. I did in fact repeatedly weigh the question, but due to the tolerant atmosphere in New York and
at the university I've described several times, I never
implemented any corresponding plans.

Nevertheless, the question hung in the air. My New
York neurologist, a colleague from New York University,
already foresaw the end of all pharmacological treatment

options. He had already begun to reduce my L-dopa dosage due to serious dyskinesias. In short video recordings of me that he and my students made, I could see for myself that my condition had deteriorated.

All of the premises that up until then had kept me from taking the initiative to undergo an operation changed after I returned to my university in Germany. Only a few weeks later, I found myself standing at the blackboard struggling to write down a few terms legibly. To this day, I recall every detail of the situation. It was a seminar on the use of the term "trauma" in the social sciences and humanities. I felt slightly dizzy and had to steady myself by holding on to the edge of the blackboard. Writing was already a problem then, but I could still manage. At that time—prior to the operation—I still had the ability to write. The larger and cruder the implement, the better. Chalk was ideal. Ballpoints and fountain pens made it difficult for me to write legibly. There was nothing to be done about it. I couldn't even write my own name legibly. Even when your hand isn't trembling or exhibiting dyskinesia, the pattern of fine motor movements we call "writing" has been destroyed.

Suddenly the dizziness became stronger. As I abruptly shifted my weight to the other leg for support, the chalk fell out of my hand. When I bent over to pick it up, I must have lurched. At any rate, in order not to fall down I had to turn toward the audience again. I saw two students imitating my bizarre body language. Perhaps they were laughing, too. Incidentally, I knew both of them and liked them quite a bit. I didn't address them. Their crimson faces betrayed their embarrassment. Their blatant contortions drove home the extent of my motor disturbances as well as the great distraction they were causing. I recalled an old neurologist's rule of thumb: when the degree of social annoyance caused by a sick person exceeds the interest in the content of his statements, he should consider withdrawing from the public. I believe that other than the three of us nobody really witnessed what transpired in that small scene. It caused no great stir when I terminated the lecture for that day. The two students disappeared immediately, and they didn't resurface during the following weeks. I would have liked to put them at rest and somewhat relieve their sense of embarrassment. If I had been able to speak with them, I would have said that experiencing annoyance in reaction to people with my symptoms is a very ancient reflex. A reflex from prehistoric times when observing every change in nature was a prerequisite for human survival. The basic anthropological configuration of human beings includes the anticipation that the movement dynamics of co-actors will conform to certain expectations, such as object constancy, predictability, and transparency with respect to a targeted goal. Those who have difficulty tolerating haphazard, exaggerated activity therefore cannot be branded cruel and coarse. It's simply that they are particularly sensitive. Within groups they often assume the role of articulating attitudes that they share with all members of the group. I myself can still recall a scene from a Parkinson's clinic where I experienced a similar impulse in rudimentary form. It was the last day of *Fasching,* the German equivalent of Carnival, and the primitive beat of the traditional songs had been drumming out of the dining room all day. At dinner, I saw a group of people dancing to the droning *Fasching* music as they headed for the table next to mine. I smiled at them self-consciously because their effusive, somewhat excessive movements embarrassed me. It was only when the music was turned off, and they nonetheless continued with their grotesque dance, that I was able to explain the situation. The people were suffering from Huntington's chorea and were gravely ill. The movements I had taken for dancing represented the victims' motor disturbances and dyskinesias.

In the evening of the same day, after the minor incident, I called a neurologist acquaintance and asked him whether he thought the operation was feasible.

9.

Deep brain stimulation (DBS) involves the implantation of electrodes in the brain through small burr holes drilled in the skull. The electrodes are regulated via an impulse generator, a kind of brain pacemaker, that is implanted underneath the clavicle. The goal is to smooth out the excessive neuronal firing in the pathological regions of the brain by sending electrical impulses through fine extensions running invisibly under the skin. In patients with Parkinson's disease, a positive effect is seen particularly in symptoms such as hypokinesia, tremor, postural and gait disturbances, exaggerated movements, and the constant fluctuation of the patients' sense of well-being. If the operation is successful, medication intake can generally be reduced by half. The particular fascination for me was the chance that I would be able to rid myself of L-dopa and therewith of my dramatic dyskinesias. One of the most drastic symptoms of late phase Parkinson's are the dyskinesias that almost all patients develop after years of taking high doses of L-dopa. It is moot to argue whether these dyskinesias are attributable to the disease or the medication. In order to ascertain that, one would either have to place a person who is seriously ill with Parkinson's on a reduced L-dopa dosage or give high doses of L-dopa to a healthy individual. Both options are out of the question.

Insights gained in recent years into the causes of Parkinson's disease have improved our understanding of the mechanism of action in DBS. It is not merely—as was previously assumed—a lack of the neurotransmitter dopamine that leads to the specific motor disturbances. In a healthy brain, a host of transmitters participate in coordinating the motor apparatus. Apparently, a dopamine deficiency disrupts the transmitter balance that nature has programmed. Nerve cells react to this with chaotic hyperactivity, and the hyperactivity causes the motor disturbances typical for the disease, such as shaking, stiffness, the slowing of all motor processes, and dyskinesias. The pacemaker, then, uses permanent electrical stimulation to deactivate the overactive nerve cells involved in the relevant regions of the brain.

Operations of this kind were first attempted in France some fifteen years ago. In the meantime, DBS has earned a reputation as an effective and proven procedure. In the summer of 2005, a major study was presented at the World Parkinson's Conference which documented the superiority of this surgical procedure in the treatment of severe Parkinson's disease with pronounced symptoms, as compared to drug therapy.

Although the procedure is considered stressful for the patient, it is not sensational in terms of medical technology. So-called "stereotactic surgery" has been performed since the beginning of the twentieth century. Initially, the term "stereotaxy" referred only to the steel ring that is screwed onto the patient's head during the operation so that he or she cannot jeopardize the outcome by moving during the procedure. DBS only became possible through dramatic advances in imaging technologies such as computer tomography and magnetic resonance imaging. Knowledge of the causes and developmental dynamics of Parkinson's and the localization of the pathological process are not new. Rather, the innovations lie in the procedures that make it possible to intervene at these locations with unprecedented precision. Deviating by even a millimeter from the pre-calculated path can turn the patient into a vegetable.

I consulted four neurologists and asked for their opinion on whether an operation was advisable in my condition. Three of them emphatically endorsed the idea, the fourth advised me against it for the time being.

Up until that time I had always thought that the selection of patients for innovative surgical techniques, where many of the outcomes and implications remained unclear, involved great social and bureaucratic efforts. My experience was different. Initially, the surgery was to be performed at the Heidelberg University Clinic; post-operative care would be handled at a clinic in the Taunus Mountains. I was confused and dismayed when I learned that there would indeed be a bed available for me at the appointed time, but that the operation itself had been postponed for six months. Within a very brief period I was able to schedule the operation at the university clinic in Cologne, where it was subsequently performed. In Cologne, of course, the surgeon cut his hand while pruning roses and to begin with had to take three weeks off. Only on the third attempt did the venture finally come to fruition.

I didn't have the impression at all times that the doctors knew what they were doing, with the exception of the central aspects of the operation. Two days prior to the surgery, I involuntarily witnessed a heated debate among younger residents over whether I was even a suitable candidate for the operation. A narrow majority was of the opinion that my Parkinson's symptoms were not grave enough to justify such a major surgical procedure. The evening before the operation, the chief surgeon came to my room and informed me that he had decided on short notice to employ a different surgical technique and to target a different region of the brain. The new method would better take into account my tendency toward depressive episodes, although it would entail the disadvantage that I would continue to be dependent on relatively high doses of Parkinson's medications after the operation. That news was very disturbing, but I was already under medication and couldn't articulate my dismay. In the morning, I was awakened by the assistant surgeon, a neurologist, who told me it had all been a misunderstanding and that the originally planned procedure would be performed.

According to the surgeons' criteria, the operation was a full success. My tremor disappeared, as well as the dyskinesias which had tormented me, particularly over the course of the previous year. My movements were fluid and relaxed. My medication intake could be drastically reduced. Today, friends who visited me in the hospital at the time tell me that I was in an outright euphoric frame of mind.

The operation was infinitely difficult. All told, it lasted almost ten hours. And the most difficult part of the procedure, drilling into the skull while it is rigidly screwed inside a stereotactic ring and one is fully conscious, must have been particularly awful. I can barely remember it. The reason that patients must remain conscious during the operation is because the neurologist assisting the surgeon must test the functionality of the stimulator while the operation is still in progress. A friend of mine told me of a telephone conversation that I apparently began while still in the best of moods. He asked me about the operation, and I described the drilling in my skull. Apparently, in order to amuse the caller and demonstrate my detachment from the event, I compared myself to a dog whose house is being attacked with a chainsaw. My speech then became unintelligible, I suddenly began to cry and simply aborted the call.

Three days after the operation, when I was already in the rehabilitation clinic, the unequivocal symptoms of trauma arose. Granted, the physicians didn't use the term, but I had read enough about post-traumatic stress reactions to understand what was going on. I was confused and tormented by severe depression. I was experiencing speech disturbances, fell down a lot, and had constant difficulty breathing. I forgot all of my telephone numbers and passwords and couldn't operate my computer anymore. My handwriting had become nothing but an illegible scrawl. The bank refused to honor my checks anymore because my signature was no longer identifiable, and I was incapable of placing a call and rectifying the situation. During my three weeks in the rehab clinic, there was little change in my condition. I quickly stopped trying to describe what I was going through to the doctors. From the time that my world shattered into pieces, I've never been in a frame of mind to complain, either because I hoped that everything would turn out all right in the end, or because I was afraid that all the dams inside of me would burst.

10

S ometimes it astonishes me that problems which are immediately evident to anyone with common sense are only acknowledged by the public when they become the subject of scientific attention. For example, the *New York Times* reported on a medical conference that focused on the dreams of patients who had survived life-threatening operations—such as open-heart surgery—or invasive brain procedures. Until then it had stood as medical dogma that when such patients were heavily sedated they were virtually unconscious and would not respond to any stimulation or to being directly addressed. The researchers discovered that it is fundamentally incorrect simply to assume that postoperative patients are in an unconscious and dreamless state. Naturally, in this group of dreamers the mind's propensity to censorship appears to be even greater than in normal dreamers. Almost half of the patients surveyed reported having nightmares. In turn, half of those patients, i.e., one quarter of the total survey population, found their dreams so unsettling that the dreams themselves became relevant medical problems. Actually, they were hardly different from post-traumatic stress symptoms. Many patients who suffered from inexplicable symptoms after their surgeries such as insomnia, lack of motivation, and depression learned only during postoperative psychotherapy to establish a connection between their operations (which were fully successful in technical respects) and their subsequent complaints. Lastly, there was the surprising finding that dreams during and after the operation differed from "normal" nightmares. Whereas nightmares exhibit an infinite range of variation depending on each dreaming subject, the postoperative dreams showed such substantial homogeneity across subjects that one could almost speak of a collective unconscious.

All post-operative dreams reflected the experience of dramatic violence; they reported murders, lynchings, mass rapes, massacres, etc.

In the first three nights at the rehabilitation clinic, I had a dream nested within a dream; the beginning and end sections overlapped so clearly it was as if my inner dream censor wanted to leave no doubt that this was one unified episode. It was a dream about a massacre in a supermarket. Even though the violence was boundless, its portrayal in the dream was still stylized. It was an ultramodern ballet. Not a movement, not a gesture, seemed coincidental. Everything served a secret choreography that had an even more nightmarish effect because there was no sound in the dream. Yet despite all this visible choreography, the silent mutual butchering didn't come across like media content; it wasn't that I was dreaming a film. I numbered among the dramatis personae in the dream, although I was not directly involved in the depicted actions themselves. I *suffered* this dream. The dream sequences themselves offered no comment or reflection on the violence they depicted. Experiencing the horror of the images was my part alone. I probably woke up screaming. As is common with nightmares, the moment the dream was finished it was recognized as a dream. That was probably also the reason why it broke off.

Ascertaining the deeper causes of the dream did not require any psychoanalytic self-exploration. Two days after the operation, I had already articulated to a friend the experience of having suffered violence, when I assumed the perspective of a dog that is compelled to live through a chainsaw attack on its dog house. It was obvious that the dream represented an attempt by my psyche to come to grips with the operation. After all, I'd never had a dream like that before, and have never had another one in the two years that have since elapsed. Perhaps this dream might also have fallen victim to the mind's censorship altogether, if its sheer dynamics and rhythmic properties hadn't burned themselves indelibly into my memory.

11

Bus No. 615 served as the shuttle between the world of clinic residents and the small town of G. Taking a taxi would have required particular chutzpah because cabs had to report to the clinic gate, and the gate attendants had instructions to scrutinize a patient's reasons for leaving the clinic, especially if the patient was new. In the clinic's own jargon, such longing to escape was ironically referred to as "hitting the road." Oftentimes it involved patients who were inclined to be confused, either due to the particular characteristics of their brain injuries or because of medication errors. Since these patients represented a particular potential for causing chaos and danger in the fussy eyes of the citizens of the small town of G., conditions at the clinic were often the subject of public attention. Hardly a week would pass where the local news sheet didn't run a report on the police bringing back a resident who had gotten away.

The police had me on their search list that morning, too, but I only discovered that after the fact.

I had lain awake since 4 A.M. listening to a CD of Verdi arias sung by the *prima donna assoluta*, Maria Callas. The arias hadn't done anything for me up until then, but that night they moved me to tears. I must have cried so hard that the night nurse became aware of me and made a jour-

nal entry on the subject. It was this journal entry as well as
the fact that I was no longer in bed and in the ward for the
first round of medication at six o'clock that set off the
alarm at the clinic.

According to the schedule, it must have been only the
second bus of the day on that cold, autumnal Sunday morning. I knew that on the tree-lined road leading to the river
the bus would pass by a house where I had lived decades
before. Those had been good times. I was probably hoping
that memories of bygone happiness would alleviate the
unhappiness that had befallen me since I became ill. I
wanted to get off at the train station, cross underneath the
tracks and—following the bus route—walk down the tree-
lined road to the river. Then I would take the bus back to
the clinic again. But as soon as I crossed underneath the
railroad tracks I was lost. An unfamiliar maze of streets
confronted me. I tortured my maltreated brain with the
absurd question of whether during the past twenty years
some dramatic world-historical events had occurred that
would have caused the streets to be renamed. I didn't have
the courage to ask directions from the increasing number
of passersby who were apparently headed for an early
mass. I was afraid of not being able to control my tears. I
was also aware of how frightening I must have looked with
my head shaved bald, white as chalk, and thick bandages
over the drill holes, like a devil who has had his horns sur-
gically removed. A female friend who had wanted to visit
me in the clinic very early that morning, finally found me
on a park bench, humming Callas arias, and returned me
to the clinic. We arrived just in time for breakfast.

Since then, I've never brooded more over any day of my
life. Certainly, it was a bad day, but that wasn't clear to me

at the time. When I spoke with friends or with my son on the telephone, I tried in vain not to make too many mistakes. My sole objective was not to be excluded from the ranks of those of sound mind by the very people who were closest to me.

I bear no grudge against the doctors who determined that I met the indications and performed the operation. In spite of all my difficulties I do not believe that they made mistakes. If one absolutely insisted on reading the story as knavery, then I was more an accomplice than the victim. My desire to be well again was so overwhelming that I would have allowed far worse things to be done to me. Nevertheless, I found the level of medical and therapeutic care so poor at the rehabilitation clinic in G., where I was transferred three days after the operation, that I certainly would have been better off without my stay in that facility.

The head physician, who was invariably very personable, wrote a kind of protocol of every visit and gave me a copy each time. As I read them, I increasingly gained the impression that the reports were discussing someone else. The conditions I had dared to mention with the greatest restraint hardly surfaced in these reports at all. For example, my desperate attempts to describe my acute shortness of breath to him and the constant, dangerous falls I took on the stairs were mentioned in a mere half-sentence, which cast doubt on my comments to boot: "The patient claims that . . . "

In an early phase of my life I was still directly influenced by an authoritarian relationship to what we sociologists today call "functional elites." Within this worldview, teachers, government personnel, even swimming pool attendants, police officers, fire fighters, the clergy, pharmacists, and likewise doctors were not simply people with a function to fulfill, and who continually had to justify themselves through the quality of the services they rendered. Instead, they were vested with a diffuse social authority that kept them relatively shielded from criticism. Happily, this authoritarian climate has changed significantly, even though one couldn't claim that, say, health care agencies have achieved the same level across the board as the institutions of performance-based society. But in our relationship to doctors, the practice of medicine, and its institutions, we patients, yours truly included, are also stuck halfway between feudal tradition and rational modernity.

Ever since I have been an adult, I've tried to ingratiate myself with doctors by attesting to the success of their therapeutic efforts, often against my better knowledge. Thus, for a long time I was assuredly a good and grateful patient. Even in the rehabilitation clinic, I was still putting up a brave front when I already knew for myself that my stay there was only making me sicker. But I was certainly a difficult patient, too. For, to the same degree that doctors are inclined toward authoritarian behavior, they themselves tend to show irrational respect toward professions and groups they perceive as superior to or even coequal with them. No other group allowed me to flaunt my professorial title as easily as physicians. A good working alliance between doctor and patient cannot come about when both parties are insecure in their own way. The physicians' insecurity increased even more when I signaled that I had become an expert in my own illness, primarily with the help of the Internet. It often occurred that by consulting the relevant American web sites, I had information on the latest developments even faster than the doctor himself.

The experience I gained in this respect after the operation only confused my views on modern medicine even further. During the next year I consulted a doctor almost every day due to a host of health problems. But I had the impression that no speech therapist, pulmonologist, psychotherapist, orthopedist, or neurologist in private practice could really help me. Some of them even candidly admitted as much. Then, during the second year after the operation, I saw hardly any doctors at all, with the exception of the essential neurological monitoring. Unfortunately, I can't claim that my problems decreased as a result, which is why I am now once again in search of doctors who are personally and professionally equal to the problems of my case.

During the weeks and months following the operation, I was often asked how I would judge the whole process on balance. It was friends who were asking the question, not the doctors who treated me. The neurosurgeon at the university clinic in Cologne never saw me again. The neurologist who assisted him during the operation and had determined that I met the indications lost all interest in me when I articulated—with great restraint at first—that I was dissatisfied with the overall outcome of the procedure. Perhaps my expectations of him were too high. One day, shortly before I left the rehab clinic, I jokingly told him that in my case the operation had merely replaced the plague with cholera. I simply had the impression that during the entire first year the upshot of this major and extremely expensive surgery had been to replace one set of grave symptoms with another. Yet I also had to admit that in general my tremor, the torturous dyskinesias, and the "off" conditions were simply gone. My medication intake had dropped by twenty-five percent. My overall mobility and endurance were markedly better than before. In contrast, I now suffered from a series of very weird and stressful symptoms, weird and stressful because my neurologist apparently also couldn't make heads or tails of the difficulties I was experiencing.

My worst post-operative symptom, which remains unchanged to this day, is a speech disturbance: my volume is too low, and my articulation is poor, slurred. Often I can't even command twenty percent of my normal speech volume. In the meantime, I discovered through my own initiative that these disturbances are due to faulty calibration of the pacemaker.

Bending over and abrupt movements cause acute shortness of breath and a fear of suffocating. Not one of the many lung specialists can tell me what causes this or even give me a name for the symptom. I can no longer form a single letter by hand. I often fall, luckily always up the stairs. Ever since the operation, my gait has become a sequence of several short, jerky steps, interrupted by constant attempts to support myself. My sense of smell and taste have disappeared almost completely.

The days I spent at the rehab clinic number among the darkest of my life. Admittedly, the profound depression of those weeks was aggravated by my physical symptoms, but it was not caused by them. Depression had established a régime of its own in my mind, one that was no longer affected by everyday joys and sorrows. Even now, after the fact, a visceral rage still comes over me when I reflect on the inferior care at that clinic. It was only shortly before my discharge that I learned of the existence of a large speech therapy department at the clinic. Immediate speech therapy intervention might have spared me the suffering I went through with my voice. There was also a psychotherapy department, whose services were virtually forced upon me. During my very first session, and without even asking me, they plastered my head—which was still shaved bald from the operation—with contacts for an electroencephalogram. They stuck me in an experimental laboratory, and I was supposed to register light stimuli that were generated by a PC. After only a few minutes, I developed a severe headache and vertigo. This treatment had no bearing on me at all, which only became clear to me through the impatient reaction of the neuropsychologist. For him I was a kind of laboratory rat. When he told me outright that he would be earning his doctoral degree based on the study in which I was a test person, without having been asked, I pulled the electrodes off my skull. From that point on he no longer greeted me.

The traditional orthopedic treatment modalities were also only used in a blanket approach, without targeting my specific symptomatology. After making several futile attempts to discuss the problems (ever since the operation!) of my extremely small-stepped gait and my tendency to fall on the stairs, I gave up and simply ignored these treatment modalities. No one was able to give me a satisfactory explanation of what therapeutic benefit would be derived in my case from playing with balls in a group and pedaling a stationary bicycle.

In spite of all my frustration and rage, as a sociologist who is fascinated by organizations I ask myself what went wrong at the clinic in G., and why the expert system of staff physicians and clinic administration did not function. In my opinion, it had nothing to do with an aggregation of individual carelessness, let alone a lack of willingness to help on the part of the personnel. The central defect of this expert system-slash-clinic lay in the inertia of institutional practices and routines that had become ingrained at some point, obscuring from view the special medical, psychological, and human aspects involved in a case. The perpetuation of institutional operating procedures had become the primary purpose, and self-replication the primary goal. Patients served merely as a means of achieving this goal.

Over the course of the two years that have elapsed since my operation, I have only gradually learned to reflect on the more general aspects of my case by drawing on information from the Internet and professional journals. There was only a modicum of comfort to be derived from my impression that I had had interesting experiences at the forefront of medical progress. The terms generally used for the electrode in my head and the pacemaker in my chest are "neuro-implant" or "neuro-enhancer." Neuro-implants are medical devices that are placed inside a person's brain and serve a wide range of therapeutic purposes. Primarily, they serve as replacements for lost or damaged neuronal functions. At present, their application is essentially limited to victims of Parkinson's disease. However, the number of applications in depressives, epileptics, and obsessive-compulsives is increasing rapidly. Critics of this development point out that widespread use of the surgical technique in Parkinson's has led to emotional changes, speech and swallowing disorders, and shallow breathing.

No data concerning frequency and intensity exists to my knowledge. Without supplying numbers, American neurological journals are reporting an increased incidence of suicides in patients with brain pacemakers. In response, a large insurance company now mandates that newly operated patients receive psychological support. Brain pacemakers are the pioneers of a trend that encompasses far more than medical applications. But even as such they are problematical—problematical due to the enormous disparity between their invasiveness, that is, the depth of penetration into the ultra complex structure of the brain, and the extensive lack of clarity on the degree of precision involved in this interaction between man and machine.

A further problem, of great concern to humanistic critics, is that, potentially, the direction is being set for a development that would lead to computer chips functioning as an interface between man and machine, thereby lending themselves as a tool to monitor and manipulate individuals and groups. This has already been in progress for a long time, for example, in the form of credit cards implanted under the skin. But even when criminologists entertain the idea of using implanted chips to track criminals, it raised the prospect of a scenario where people are turned into remote-controlled robots.

The *New York Times* reported on a conference where neuro-scientists and philosophers discussed the social ramifications of improved medications for the brain. For example, Ritalin—a medication that alleviates severe attention disorders in children—came under discussion. Also debated was a soon-to-be released drug for Alzheimer's disease, which promises to improve memory enormously. If these medications, among which we can also count the new potency drugs, the new class of antidepressants, and also brain pacemakers, were unambiguously and exclusively remedies for the sick, they wouldn't pose a problem. But there *is* a problem because these new therapeutic tools blur the classical demarcation between "sick" and "healthy." The tremendous media attention these drugs are receiving is in itself an indication that the pharmaceutical industry has targeted a larger group of consumers than those who have been clearly identified as neurologically ill. Rather, the drugs are directed at an infinitely larger market consisting of those who are dissatisfied with their performance, be it their memory, their sexual potency, their mood, etc. "Neuro-enhancement" is the term commonly used in professional circles for these supports, which, as byproducts of neurological research, can also help healthy people to better master their lives.

Which rationale and authority should public officials invoke to forbid the consumption of Ritalin, Prozac, or Viagra as aids that help people cope with their lives? The case would be clear-cut only if the new medications were accompanied by serious side effects. Then, precisely defined medical indications alone would justify buying them. Fundamentalist critics of this development still maintain that the integrity of human nature generates health through its own vital energy. It reminds one of the romantic critics who faulted industrial civilization based on a comparison with a *natura naturans*, a prehistorical world still devoid of technological development. But just like the external nature that surrounds us, our bodies contain no natural essence that is untainted by technological intervention and could serve as a clear criterion to distinguish between healthy and sick. We ourselves do not deserve the credit for our own health. A small survey conducted on a randomly selected group of, say, fifty-year-olds, would show that under the medical conditions prevailing in pre-industrial society only a fraction of this group would still be alive. Thus, in order to deny healthy people access to the means of improving their lives, one would have to invoke an ability to distinguish clearly between healthy and sick, and that doesn't exist. Even those who are healthy are only well to the extent that they have access to medical technology.

Yet what kind of consequences would it entail if access to so-called neuro-enhancers were expanded far beyond the circle of those with medical indications, to include anyone who could pay for them and simply wanted to have a better quality of life? That would undermine a fundamental differentiation upon which the notion of justice in our society is founded, so to speak. For centuries not only the field of philosophy but also many constitutions and legal texts have differentiated between two forms of inequality: natural differences and social inequality. As natural beings, we differ with respect to gender, skin color, physical strength, etc. As social beings, we are unequal according to social status, high or low class, rich or poor, etc. The doctrine or ideology of achievement-based society alleges that a just society is possible. The more faithfully the existing social differences reflect the actual distribution of talent, strength, and achievement motivation, the more just the society.

Meanwhile, this traditional differentiation encountered difficulties when it came to attributing such capacities to individuals. Are individuals the legitimate proprietors of their memory or their capabilities? The modern age has seen differing opinions on this very subject. Conservatives were inclined to attribute differences in ability and achievement to a person's innate natural endowment. "The Left" viewed these inequalities as a product of society, as the result of material living conditions, social opportunities, child raising styles, etc.

If, however, specific individual capabilities are increasingly no longer nature's dowry, but rather the discrete consequences of medical technology, then the distinction between natural and social inequality no longer applies—with unforeseeable consequences.

12.

I n November, after I had more or less fled the clinic, I
drove to my house in Tuscany. I had bought it almost
twenty years before with my partner, the mother of my
son. During the final nights in the clinic, as the lonely
screaming of a female patient and the voices inside of me
kept sleep away, I would remember the call of the little owl
and the song of the nightingale and felt the desire to be
alone there. My friends were against the trip. They would
have preferred to see me in Frankfurt in a supervised living community. But my intuition was correct: the breach
between the world and me, which had grown even wider
at the clinic, could only be repaired in solitude. Naturally,
my aloneness was not absolute. A Spanish tour guide and
his adopted Moroccan daughter lived in the building next
door, and in another building a man lived who raised the
exclusive Sienese breed of pigs. I barely exchanged words
with them, nor did I feel much like talking. It was as if the
disturbances in my language center affected different lan-
guages in different ways. I could still speak impeccable,
fluent English, while speaking my own native language
was torture. My Italian, which was passable at one time,
had been virtually obliterated.

The concerns of my friends were not completely
unfounded. Not that I was in danger of committing sui-

cide. The movies in my head, in particular my dreams at night, were far too exciting for me to feel any desire to terminate them. I was merely extremely physically weak and had the disastrous tendency to fall upstairs, especially when I was carrying baggage. But it seems I must always have been very relaxed when I fell. The stairs in the house in Tuscany were the only place I once bloodied my head.

I had been lying awake since five o'clock, watching the light behind the shutters become brighter and brighter. Only a few hours before I had downed a bottle of red wine and taken a bromazepam. After a few hours of unconsciousness, I was awake again, alert and empty at the same time. The only thing I could remember at first was the impression I'd had falling asleep, namely, that my world had broken into pieces ever since the operation, and that I would no longer have the strength and energy to piece it back together again. I finally got up and opened the shutters in order to chase away the morning twilight.

The deep blue sky was crisscrossed by the contrails of high-altitude fighter jets heading for their air base in Grosseto. With the sun shining on their silvery bodies, they could have been fish that had fallen from space.

Seen in retrospect, and probably also from the perspective of my experience, I would not have been able to say how I was actually doing. My inclination to stare silently and rigidly straight ahead could have been an acute depression, for which I would have had every justification. After all, not only had the operation failed to fulfill my hopes for a new life, I was forced to admit to myself that, all in all, I was in worse condition than before. Yet I wasn't dejected or sad or even angry with my doctors. A hitherto unknown indifference had taken possession of me, an equanimity that might also have resulted from a meditative exercise. I constantly had to think of a saying hanging in a simple frame on the wall of the first class waiting room at the Frankfurt train station: "There's nothing in the world that can replace your peace of mind." I had my peace of mind, but it was the foul peace following a lost war. The things of life had lost their savor and color. At eight o'clock in the evening I dropped into bed with my clothes on and fell into an exhausted sleep for several hours, until the clammy cold woke me up again. I was still feeding the stove with logs long after midnight, again trying to fall asleep; generally I didn't succeed. Then at about four I got up, took a long hot shower, and in the pale early morning light drove down completely empty roads to places where I had occasionally been happy in earlier days. First, there were the natural springs at Petriolo. The name doesn't promise much, but Petriolo is a magical place. All of the pre-Christian civilizations left their traces here. After waging battle, warriors came here to tend their wounds. Today, miraculous curative powers are still attributed to the radioactive sulfur mud. And even now, shortly before sunrise, the citizens of the surrounding villages were arriving to rub the healing mud onto their old legs, seamed with veins, and their rheumatic limbs. The population ensured the preservation of the elaborate system of bathing pools, which are arranged in tiers like an amphitheater and extend down to the river.

In the early-morning hours I was usually the only person in the water. Stretched out in a warm pool, I thought of many a Friday evening I spent here in the summer of 1990. The view that presented itself from the bridge had a fairy-tale quality back then. Scattered campfires were already burning. The moon had risen. Stars sparkled in the sky. Later, they were joined by fireflies, and after midnight by myriads of shooting stars. Weekends were party time in Petriolo. Blankets lay spread on the small beach between the cold river and the hot sulfur water, illumined by the flickering light of torches and the fires. Children ran back and forth, dogs barked. People were passing around bottles and joints. Now it was quiet and cold and foggy.

Another magical place was San Galgano. San Galgano is a late-Gothic church ruin situated alone on a high plateau and surrounded by scattered farmsteads. Originally, only the roof was damaged. But several years of rain and winter storms removed what remained of it, followed by the interior plaster, and brought down part of the exterior walls. The latter have been reconstructed of simple brick. Here, too, I was entirely by myself because it was early on a cold November morning. The first times I re-visited San Galgano, I was overwhelmed by memories of the time before I became ill. For example, I recalled a concert on an August night in the late eighties. Because my son was little, I didn't enter the performance hall, i.e., the nave of the church, but listened to the concert from the outside. I was lying, with the child asleep on my arm, in front of an empty window opening where a large heap of white marble gravel had been piled up. There was a full moon. Stars were twinkling. After the tenth meteorite I stopped making wishes. It was always the same wish: that things would always stay that way.

My son was ten the first time he asked me what it's actually like to get older, "to be on the downhill slope of life."

Even then, he sensed that there was more to being grown-up than enjoying the freedoms denied children. With the onset of puberty, it dawned on him that the end of childhood spelled the beginning of a risky situation which, aside from all gains in autonomy, can also be determined by misfortune, failure, sickness, and death. All of the fears people have when they are young come true over the course of a lifetime. Parents and friends die. Partnerships break up. One fails to reach the goals one has set. All health care and medical technology notwithstanding, death steals its way into life like water that seeps into the cracks of a stone and then breaks it apart in the winter. And yet, paradoxically, one still has the experience that everything is not as bad as one thought. Not in the sense of a frivolous, "Hurray, I'm still alive," but in the sense of experiencing an adventurous journey within one's own soul, one's own body. Within one's self.

13.

I consistently shunned the company of Parkinson's sufferers. In places where contact was unavoidable, such
as neurological clinics and waiting rooms, I always
acted as if I weren't one of them. The forced cheerfulness
found in self-help groups was particularly offensive.
Granted, I had a burning interest in the patients' histories—for example, how dramatically their Parkinson's was
progressing, how long they had been sick, which medications they took and how much. But I just had the completely unsubstantiated impression that the people who
gather in self-help groups have nothing in common other
than their little, unwelcome secrets.

As a result, I was extremely reserved when I made the
acquaintance of Stefan through the offices of a colleague.
Stefan was several years older than I and generally ahead
of me in many respects. His field was physics, a hard,
clear science that I greatly admired. Stefan was also seven
years ahead of me in terms of symptom development. He
was having a difficult time; his wife had left him. At the
time I met him he was just retiring. I think he was being
forced to leave. He spoke so softly and indistinctly that he
could no longer be understood in a lecture hall. His
tremor was so pronounced that he spilled food on himself
when he ate, like a little child. I registered all of this with

the cold precision of a public health officer. Meanwhile, what I found deeply shocking and heartrending was a trait I had already noticed in myself: the complete absence of all cheerfulness, all optimism. He created the impression of a person under a mountain of sandbags, desperately trying to free himself with the sole hand that was still sticking out.

Stefan was a wretched figure, although I never heard him complain. He was a portent for me, the handwriting on the wall. The interest that we soon developed in one another was imbalanced. We were united by a diagnosis. We were separated by the course of the disease. I wouldn't call it a friendship. He roped me in as a co-victim; I viewed his poor condition as proof that I had nothing in common with him other than a poor prognosis.

We agreed on only one point and didn't tire of discussing it: our mixture of dread and despair in the face of a future we already knew would be ghastly. It moved me almost to tears when he told me that all he wanted was to wake up lighthearted one more time so that he could look forward to the day, to seeing a woman or a friend—just for the fun of it.

I recall one conversation in particular. We were sitting in a glass-enclosed patio at the clinic early one afternoon. Lunch was over, and the patients filed past us on the way to their rooms. Without exception, they were elderly, stooping, and miserable, hardly any of them without an aid such as a cane or a rollator walker; some were in wheelchairs. At that, Stefan raised the topic of suicide.

He spoke softly but his enunciation was clear as glass. I understood every word. He did not harbor any immediate intention of killing himself, but during the recent weeks he had thought a lot about "voluntary death." He said he wasn't desperate enough yet to take that final step. He merely wanted to reclaim authority over his own life. Only if his life was completely devoid of joy, or devoid of the possibility of determining where and when he found joy, he would resort to suicide. He offered me a pact, a reciprocal service based on friendship. He wanted me to enter into a covenant that I would tell him when the time had come. And he pledged to do the same for me. In his opinion, overlooking that point in time was the actual object of his fear. I didn't feel comfortable with the conversation and have successfully avoided him ever since. For me, his offer of a pact crossed a line. I want to live.

14

All my life I've had secrets. The first may well have their origins in the sexual awakening of early puberty. I had just turned twelve, and for a long time I believed that nocturnal emissions and the technique of producing them were exclusively my experience. Nevertheless, I must have sensed that performing this activity was taboo, otherwise I would have simply asked a friend or my father. At the end of childhood, masturbation was my first secret. The second was serious acne on my chest and back. From the age of thirteen to twenty-one, no one, with the exception of a dermatologist and the panel that performed my military induction examination, had ever seen my scarred torso naked. At age forty-six I learned that I had Parkinson's disease. I kept it a secret for many years; now I can no longer conceal it. Now I walk through the streets and count the oncoming pedestrians who look at my asymmetrical, shuffling gait with curiosity or alienation. It was a key theme in my life that other people were not allowed to know things. Almost every relationship I had with a woman was defined by a secret that I either kept from her or which we kept from the rest of the world. A relationship where the innermost motives were completely transparent for both partners as well as for the world was utterly foreign to me. Not that I wouldn't have wanted one, but a powerful neurotic dynamic prevented it. I was always convinced that divulging the secret would completely discredit me in the eyes of the world and those who were close to me. I wasted a large portion of my time and vital energy shielding my secrets from discovery. This activity was so central to me that it was not limited to individual aspects of keeping the respective secrets but consolidated into an attitude, a *habitus* where I would act cautiously, like an agent behind enemy lines, and play my cards close to the chest. For that reason, I could never understand the enthusiasm of cell phone users for being reachable anywhere, by anyone, at all times. But part of this disposition is a culture of lying. It wasn't that I simply withheld parts of the truth, but that I already lied far in advance. In my case, a question such as exactly when I had arrived or when I would be leaving again never stood a chance of receiving a truthful answer. For me, not having to tell the truth was a prerequisite for freedom. Because of that, I never had a guilty conscience about it. After all, these were not lies aimed at obtaining selfish advantages, but rather at protecting myself from the world's passion for control which, I believed, required my constant vigilance.

This is the thirteenth year that I've had Parkinson's, and for some time the obviousness of my symptoms has forced me to reveal my secret, perhaps the biggest secret of my life. For example, every so often I manage to begin a major public lecture with a reference to my illness. On those occasions, I relate how I register during my lectures that the attention of the audience focuses on my symptoms instead of the content of my talk. Whenever I find the courage to mention my illness, I am heaped with praise after the lecture. Many people seem to sense how dearly it costs me to reveal my secret. Indeed, it's tremendously difficult for me to utter the word "Parkinson's" in public. I continue to feel ill at ease. Actually, I'd like just the lecture to be appreciated, without any notice of the lecturer. What receives recognition, however, is the courage I show in making my condition known, while other victims of disease hide from the world. A secret is the private obverse of a so-called stigma.

In our everyday usage, the term "stigma" refers to a physical defect that prevents the person who bears it from participating fully in social interactions. Etymologically, the word derives from the Greek. It referred to non-reversible physical characteristics that revealed something potentially discrediting about the moral status of the person who bore them. To ensure that no mistakes arose, and to prevent all attempts at deception or concealment by the bearer of the stigma, the individual was additionally branded with a mark or scarred with cuts and thereby marked as a slave, criminal, enemy of the polis, etc. In the Christian tradition, this barbaric ancient custom and its meaning were reversed into something positive. For example, in early Christianity scars were viewed as a sign of having been chosen by God, as an indication that the person who bore the wounds was already in a state of grace. In modern usage the term is once again applied descriptively to physical anomalies. Naturally, "stigma" is now a negative term. Those who use it—for example, in special education—do so in an attempt to criticize prevailing practices of stigmatization. The target of the criticism is the still widespread practice of using visible physical defects as a reason to deny full participation in the social communications process to those who are affected.

Thus, the inclination to stigmatize people implies classifying them in a discrediting social category and branding them with the defects they would otherwise keep secret. Simply entreating people to encounter others without prejudice masks the degree that our inclination to stigmatize is linked to the basic structure of social perception. In routine contacts this is unproblematic. In daily life we frequent social spaces such as school, the workplace, public offices, etc., which determine in a quasi natural way the circle of people we meet in them. It's completely different when we encounter strangers. For example, if we're walking in the woods on a foggy autumn day, we only see people coming toward us as blurs. Nevertheless, the moment we make visual contact a rudimentary categorization process begins. The people's movement patterns, their physical bearing, the volume of their voices, their clothing, are registered with amazing precision. This hectic process of social categorization only settles down when our search for any stigma has yielded results. For example, when we believe we can determine that the people are drunk, or that they are a group of school children who have lost their way, or perhaps escaped convicts, etc. Often, we have an opportunity to cross-check the validity of our attributions against reality, although frequently we don't do so, and content ourselves with the prejudice. Which is not to say that stigmas exist only in the imagination of the prejudiced. On the contrary, they are extremely real. In social psychology we differentiate between three groups of "stigmas": first, physical deformaties; second, character weaknesses and conspicuous behavior; and third, the so-called phylogenetic stigmas of ethnic and religious background.

Most recently, criticism of this widespread practice, particularly of stigmatizing certain groups of patients, is consolidating into outright de-stigmatization movements. Although generally seen in major US cities, there are in the meantime also large-scale sports events organized by volunteers in European urban centers. These de-stigmatization initiatives began as events that are open to the general public ("Run for the Cure") and involve fundraising for research on life-threatening diseases. But that's not all. A far more important secondary aspect is to create public acceptance for handicaps. Handicap is the term used to deal with disability in a non-stigmatizing form.

Naturally, the growing criticism of the practice of stigmatization lacks a philosophical foundation. The vast importance of the concept of stigmatization within day-to-day social perception is an expression of a well-nigh social Darwinist view of human communication. Every interaction sequence between two people represents a re-negotiation: who bears the stigma, and who is the warrantor of normality and entitled to the privilege of judging his fellow human beings.

In the modern age, discourse on physical disability, insanity, and illness is guided by a binary schematic of normal versus abnormal. This perception is so deep-seated that even the pioneers of the de-stigmatization movements can conceive of improvement only in the form of more liberal regulations for dealing with stigmatization.

The flippancy with which normal people are assigned stigmatizing labels for minor annoyances points to the almost anthropological substrate of this behavior.

Meanwhile, a different kind of behavior, a different model of behavior is obviously indicated and recommends itself on the strength of the large number of stigmatized individuals alone. If everyone, or at least almost everyone, were to number among the stigmatized at least once in his or her life, this factum could stand as a *humanum*, a quintessential core experience of human life. This would correspond to an anthropology where fragility, vulnerability, and affliction with a stigma become the criteria for belonging to the human race.

15.

The worst side effect of the operation was the disruption of the speech center in my brain. It was particularly depressing that the speech disturbances were gradually increasing. In the rehabilitation clinic I did not yet grasp the full extent of this. Diagnosing speech disturbances is difficult. They find no mention in my doctor's reports. Also, speech disturbances can't be identified with the precise objectivity of a computer program. As a general rule, we all speak colloquially. Colloquial usage is defined by deviations from proper grammar and the phonetic structure of standard pronunciation. Most Parkinson's sufferers are old, they often speak in dialect and are retired. It only became clear to me after a year, when I had returned to work, that if the speech disturbances continued I would have to retire. True, speech disturbances were mentioned during the preliminary discussions leading up to the operation, but the doctors were convinced that they were a transient problem, a side effect. I was confronted with the first dramatic manifestation of this side effect in the rehabilitation clinic, on the fourth day after my operation. The management of the clinic offered patients the option of storing their cash and credit cards in a safe. At certain scheduled times one could withdraw the amounts required for day-to-day life in the clinic. When the time came, I entered the cashier's office with self-confidence and the habitual aplomb one inevitably acquires in conjunction with a successful life and the linguistic competence that can be summoned at any time. But as I confronted the impatient and impolite administrator, I was unable to remember my own name. That marked the beginning of a series of word-finding difficulties that plagued me particularly when I faced people who weren't able to put themselves into my position. Although these symptoms subsided three weeks later, they laid the foundation for a multitude of vague speech impairments that continue to this day. My speech is soft and "washed out." The better part of all my attempts to establish contact and communicate fail because, all conscious effort notwithstanding, I can't speak loudly or clearly enough. Particularly burdensome for me and alienating for those in my environment is my pronounced stuttering. For situations that require me to speak in public, I have mental lists of words that are just too much for my tongue: Mexico City, identity, in the middle, etc. Before the lecture, I practice those words particularly or substitute others that are easier to pronounce. If I'm before a familiar audience, and one of those special words refuses allegiance but is key to the lecture, I resort to self-irony and refer to the forbidding word by its initial letter. Thus, the word "globalization" simply becomes the "G-word."

Since my speech is not only washed out and poorly articulated, but also very soft, I use an expensive amplifier, even in small seminar rooms. Nevertheless, over the past year it has happened increasingly often that even using an amplifier couldn't prevent me from becoming so exhausted in less than an hour that I wasn't able to speak at all.

The specific speech disturbances that emerged after the operation in my case correspond with those that many Parkinson's sufferers develop in the late stage of their illness—without having the operation. This confusing state of affairs is also discussed in the professional literature on postoperative management of deep brain stimulation. Indeed, the physicians and speech therapists I consulted after the operation also tended to classify the disturbances as typical for Parkinson's and to advise me to accept the symptoms just as I had learned to tolerate the other impairments of the disease. But I refused to accept the disturbances because they had only appeared *after* the operation.

For those who are affected, speech disturbances are so dramatic because they represent a stigma that has an immediate and permanently discrediting effect. I have often experienced embarrassment when I was simply unable to communicate a certain message during a meeting because I stuttered and shied at a certain word, like a horse in front of an obstacle. The stigmatizing effect of speech disturbances is symptomatic for the value our society places on verbal communication and communicative competence. A paraplegic in a wheelchair who has command of everyday speech doesn't create nearly as much collective discomfort at a public gathering as a stutterer, even though the paraplegic's handicap is far more visible and grave.

The worst thing about these disturbances is that consequences result from their duration alone. I've been living with them for two years now, but they don't remain on the surface of the personality like a wart or a visible scar. In order to prevent it from becoming obvious to the world that the vocabulary I can use without difficulty is shrinking, I unconsciously limit myself to the words I can master without any problems. I'm afraid that my ability to articulate is falling ever more markedly behind my thinking, concept formation, and power of reasoning. This confronts me with the perverse options of either falling silent in public or continuing to speak until my audience no longer wants to listen.

One year after the operation, a light appeared in the tunnel of uncertainty when a neurologist at a different clinic suggested simply turning off the pacemaker as an experiment. It was as if I were channeling a spirit. That very second my voice returned, sonorous and clearly enunciated, only slightly hoarse. Interestingly, not only was my speech immediately functional in a technical sense, but my intellectual activity and cognitive faculties were quite literally switched on again. During the fifteen minutes that we turned off the device, it was as if a PC were booting up in my head, and its clicking and whirring were signaling that my brain was working.

Simply leaving the unit turned off didn't seem like a viable solution to us. After all, it was to be expected that the other parameters of my mental condition would rapidly deteriorate. The experience of turning off the pacemaker, together with reading hundreds of documents online pertaining to postoperative management of deep brain stimulation (DBS), gave me reason to assume that my problems after the operation could be traced to a setting of the electrode in my head that was creating an ongoing disturbance of the brain's language center. The neurologist and a manufacturer's representative began trying to find settings that took my clinical picture into account. Unfortunately, the two of them did not succeed in finding a mid-range setting that would have allowed me to live well. They confirmed my suspicion that one of the two electrodes was irritating a section of the brain that was functionally responsible for speech. Yet they were able to help me in a different problem area. Within one second, a small change in the voltage and a simple polarity reversal of the electrodes in my head improved the massive depression I had been experiencing for a year. I was both fascinated and frightened that the depression fell away from me just like that, as if an iron band around my soul had snapped. The very ease of the process intrigued me. The press of a button, confirmed through a barely audible digital beep and supported by a tiny LED, and my overcast skies instantly cleared. The friends I called thought I had just fallen in love, that's how happy I must have sounded.

Frightening and also somehow humiliating was the banality of the process. I had felt the weight of the world in the innumerable sorrowful tales that had gone through my head that year. Simply to wipe it all away at the push of a button seemed almost frivolous. Maybe it would be fitting at this point to differentiate: we distinguish between endogenous and exogenous depression. The latter entails a deep sense of sadness caused, say, by the death of someone we are close to. It usually has a rationally understandable onset. When life changes, then the depression abates, too. This kind of sorrow is at best a sub-clinical symptom, although it can precipitate a structural, i.e., endogenous depression. Endogenous depressions are physical illnesses and are generally caused by neurotransmitter dysfunctions which are independent of external events. Yet these clinical depressions also have their material aspects, expressing themselves, for example, in apathy or a lack of motivation lasting for years. I am deeply convinced that diagnostic differentiation between the two conditions is possible. Parkinson's sufferers are familiar with both. Thus, the accusation that it is frivolous to make depression disappear by simply pressing a button can only apply to exogenous depression, because only in such cases is it possible that one would be swindled out of the fruits of one's arduous grieving efforts.

For some time, I've had a regulator that allows me to adjust my pacemaker amplitudes on my own, according to a scale prescribed by my doctor. Depending on whether I need to walk for some distance or speak in public, I have to enter commands into my pacemaker much the way I would on my computer. If I want to enunciate clearly, I have to set the amplitude very low, which then regularly leads to relative immobility and depression. If I want to walk for more than half a kilometer, I have to set the level correspondingly high, which then makes me speak inaudibly and sound washed out. I can't talk while I walk.

Several months ago, I traveled to New York with my son, who is now twenty-one. The trip was meant as a journey of reconciliation for the two of us. I agreed to the trip even though I was convinced that the conflict we wanted to eliminate once and for all could basically only be contained, but not resolved.

My son is extremely articulate, which gives him a degree of communicative competence that absolutely intimidates me since I partially lost my own speaking competence. He took exception to personality changes which (in his opinion) had resulted from my illness. Particularly in reaction to my restricted ability to speak—compared to my previous mode of existence as an intellectual with a powerful command of the language—I had to a large extent withdrawn from the social world. Even the numerous unavoidable social contacts within the framework of my professional activities proved overwhelming for me. I simply no longer had the desire to be subjected even in my personal life to the same stress I regularly experienced in public as a person stigmatized by serious illness. My son argued that this tendency to fall silent and retreat from life reflected a deep character disposition in me. It was in his opinion highly advisable for me to resist this tendency with the utmost resolution, particularly since my illness was encouraging my inclination toward depressive withdrawal from the world. The worst suspicion he expressed was that I was using my illness as a tool to keep responsibilities and demands at bay which I was simply too lethargic or frightened to fulfill.

In numerous conversations with my son as well as with friends who knew both of us, his position became clearer to me. I had always been inclined to perceive his position in this conflict as that of an adult, and precisely *not* that of a child or a son. If anyone else had accused me of exploiting my illness, I would have been completely justified in refusing to tolerate such unfair meddling in a life that simply had to be judged by special standards. My son, however, as my son, has every right in the world to demand that I, as his father, assume responsibility for myself in my relationship with him. This legitimate expectation is built into the father-son constellation. It cannot be ignored without seriously hurting the child.

Meanwhile, conversations were not the only place where this became clear to me. Seen from without, it was an unimportant event that helped me gain clarity. But for symbolical reasons that only I myself could fully grasp, it was perhaps the most important event after the operation.

A friend of mine in New York, a female colleague whom I had called to arrange a get-together during the few days we would be spending there, invited me to a dinner at the Columbia University Faculty Club. I knew this kind of event from earlier times. A colleague presents a short lecture on the occasion of the publication of a new book manuscript. A formidable dinner is served beforehand. The lecture and the dinner are by invitation. Surrounding a core group of permanent participants, there is a fluctuating circle of guests who receive invitations in a separate ceremonial. Such invitations are a great honor and it behooves the invitee to participate actively in the discussion. My colleague wanted to do me a special favor with the invitation, and since I didn't want to hurt her feelings I initially accepted. My illness, I thought to myself, would supply an excuse to liberate me at short notice from my voluntary commitment. But I had forgotten to factor my son into the calculation. By coincidence, he was present and asked my colleague whether he could come along. He was going to be studying at an English university in the upcoming term and took a keen interest in this example of Anglo-Saxon academic culture. He, too, was invited, and if I were now to decline the invitation despite my initial acceptance, it would have been particularly rude. I had already written a monograph on the topic of the evening. It had also been published in English, so I was on a sure footing for the obligatory discussion.

After a festive dinner we were ushered into a small auditorium where the function took place. The seminar followed a certain academic liturgy. Since the lecture had already been sent to the participants beforehand, the speaker was brief. In the first round of discussion, each participant had to respond to the lecture with a five-minute position statement. In addition, guests were expected to introduce themselves in detail. The seating arrangement was favorable for me: I would be the last person called upon to speak in the first round. When the first participant began, my son briefly leaned over to me and said almost inaudibly, "You've got to speak here. You can't dodge this one, I'd be mortified."

It was only then that naked fear gripped me. Matthias Claudius said, "In danger and in great need, the middle course leads to death." It occurred to me that as I was packing my backpack for the long subway ride from Washington Square up to Columbia, I had wondered why I'd brought the clunky gray control unit for my pacemaker along on the trip. Almost a year had passed since my session with the neurologist who had suggested just turning the unit off every once in a while. I had on occasion lowered the amplitude of the remote control and thereby achieved modest gains in my ability to speak, although I had never had the courage simply to turn the thing off. And yet, that's exactly what I now did, about ten minutes before it would be my turn in the sequence of speakers. I willfully accepted the possibility that this might make me collapse or experience an attack of weakness. Even that would have been better than making unintelligible, poorly articulated comments in a feeble voice.

It went well. Actually, it came off brilliantly, even

though I was somewhat hoarse. At least for the ten or so minutes that I spoke, I was my old self again with the physical and intellectual ability that had been at my command before the operation. Since I was so afraid of undesirable side effects, I turned the unit on again after my short presentation. Even my son didn't notice anything. But when I was done speaking he whispered, "That was really great. You see, you can do it after all."

I was overcome with wild joy, dampened only by the sadness that I couldn't really share it with anyone. The possibility of turning off the pacemaker's remote control for a time, at the touch of a button, and enabling myself to speak as clearly and succinctly as before, ensured that I could retain my job and restored my pride and professional authority. Naturally, in the screeching subway my son asked me why I had suddenly been able to hold forth the way I'd been known to speak in earlier days. When I disclosed the infinitely trivial reason, he just silently shook his head. To this day I don't know whether he believed me. I wouldn't hold it against him if he didn't. Certain things are just too grotesque for one to insist that others accept as true. The next day I contacted a representative of the manufacturer, as well as four neurologists I knew, to inquire whether occasionally turning the device off could do me any harm. None of them could answer my question.

Technology critic Ivan Illich formulated a basic criterion that allows us to determine the benefit of any technical invention. He subsumes the criterion under the concept of "conviviality." The German equivalent of the word would be "Lebensdienlichkeit," that is, "of service in life." A technical invention is to be welcomed if it increases people's ability to act, while still allowing them the freedom to determine its use. For Illich, the telephone is a positive example. One can use the telephone to arrange a rendezvous or to craft a conspiracy against a political opponent. The invention of the automobile is an thoroughly different story. In the early years, cars may still have contributed to the mobility of those who used them. But the more they became the core element of a new transportation system, the more the means turned into the end. The heavier the traffic, the more slowly cars can be driven. A system of asphalt and concrete roads now deforms nature, which had previously been intact. The economy becomes dependent on a production dynamic where the manufacture and sale of automobiles gradually turn into the most important parameters of the entire national economy.

Most of Ivan Illich's books discuss the topic of the medical-industrial complex. According to his theory, the very industry whose products and institutions are supposed to correspond to people's life interests, is the least convivial. Now, these books were written in the '70s and '80s of the previous century. It would be interesting to know how he would have assessed the more recent development of neural-prosthetics and neuro-enhancers. The fact that the potential pool of customers will exceed by far the number of those who fit the definition of sick, and that the potential for social control will be many times larger than with customary technologies, would only seem to corroborate Illich's theory.

I was able to experience the potential for social control through pacemaker technology on my own person. The neurologist who was treating me pointed out the noticeable effect the electronics had produced through my new, self-confident use of the pacemaker.

The greater ability to exert control in social situations that is associated with the new freedom in the use of a pacemaker has one disadvantage: an ever increasing number of intimate, spontaneous reactions begin to be possible solely through the agency of the control unit. Granted, I am once again able to deliver a lecture, but even during the discussion I have to turn the unit off again because I'm inundated by waves anxiety, depression, and difficulty breathing. The worst part of my new condition is being ashamed in society that my human communications are being mediated by a piece of equipment. More and more often it's being pointed out to me how creepy (to quote a female friend) the technology used in my case must seem to the naïve mind. Long-term medication use will turn a person with a neurological illness into a zombie, a pacemaker turns him into a Frankenstein.

If there were only some reliable way to improve my condition—to achieve an improvement that doesn't have to be acquired at the cost of new drawbacks.

N ear the exit for Friedberg the valley carved into the Taunus hills widens into the Rhine-Main plain. In the distance one sees the skyline of Frankfurt, embedded in a panorama of small parks and postmodern industrial buildings. I was still feeling the shock of my collision with the truck. I would have liked to be driving slower, especially since the remains of my side mirror were still attached by two spiral wires and the oncoming wind was rhythmically knocking it against the body of my car. But I was surrounded by vehicles that were all driving very fast, as if they were attracted to the scent of the nearby city. In the meantime, dusk had turned into the still-light darkness of an early summer evening. When the heavy traffic finally gave me an opening, I switched into the right lane and headed for the Taunus-blick rest stop, where I parked my car between the huge, dark trucks. In the twilight of the parking-lot lights, and with their roaring refrigeration units, they seemed like a herd of primeval monsters. Using a pair of pliers I separated the wrecked mirror from the body of the car.

Over the last few months I have tried—with some success—to secure the positive stocks of my life rather than lament what I am no longer able to have or to do. Thus, I have begun to reconcile myself with my pacemaker. It gives me energy and mobility. I can accept it now because I more often take the liberty of turning it off. Then I can think, talk and formulate thoughts as I speak, just like before, as if nothing had ever happened—although only for two hours.

After much training I am now capable of walking for two hours. I have my medication regimen under control. New medications will appear on the market and relieve the dizziness that often plagues me. Of course, I must resign myself to being viewed as handicapped. This, in turn, is bearable because many people show me that they like me and thereby convey a more positive self-image to me than I had before my illness. And I have begun to follow PD research on the Internet, again. Just as deep brain stimulation gripped my attention several years ago, it is now spheramine, a magical word that reminds one of precious stones. This involves the implantation of human retinal tissue into the putamen area of the brain, which promises a more effective treatment of PD.

I do not know whether I can still reckon with a significant improvement of my symptoms—someday. But I don't want to stop dreaming about the things I will eventually be able to do again: walk through large crowds of people without fear, dance, talk with strangers in noisy train stations, stroll along the path that leads from Harlem down to Battery Park on a sunny September day in New York.

The preconditions and consequences of all the important decisions in life are too complex for the individuals involved to be fully aware of them. That should not offend our narcissism in any way. On the contrary, one of the prerequisites for happiness is realizing life's open-endedness and having an inkling that beyond the next mountain range, around the next bend in the road, lies an unknown land.

About the Author

Helmut Dubiel studied German literature and philosophy at the Universities of Bielefeld and Bochum. He was a visiting professor at UC Berkeley and New York University from 1998 to 2002, before returning to his position as professor of sociology at the University of Giessen, where he has taught since 1992. In 1982, at the age of forty-six, he was diagnosed with Parkinson's Disease.

Carmine Abate
Between Two Seas
"A moving portrayal of generational continuity."—*Kirkus*
192 pp • $14.95 • 978-1-933372-40-2

Salwa Al Neimi
The Proof of the Honey
"Al Neimi announces the end of a taboo in the Arab world:
that of sex!"—*Reuters*
160 pp • $15.00 • 978-1-933372-68-6

Alberto Angela
A Day in the Life of Ancient Rome
"Fascinating and accessible."—*Il Giornale*
392 pp • $16.00 • 978-1-933372-71-6

Muriel Barbery
The Elegance of the Hedgehog
"Gently satirical, exceptionally winning and inevitably
bittersweet."—Michael Dirda, *The Washington Post*
336 pp • $15.00 • 978-1-933372-60-0

Stefano Benni
Margherita Dolce Vita
"A modern fable...hilarious social commentary."—*People*
240 pp • $14.95 • 978-1-933372-20-4

Timeskipper
"Benni again unveils his Italian brand of magical realism."—*Library Journal*
400 pp • $16.95 • 978-1-933372-44-0

Massimo Carlotto
The Goodbye Kiss
"A masterpiece of Italian noir."—*Globe and Mail*
160 pp • $14.95 • 978-1-933372-05-1

Death's Dark Abyss
"A remarkable study of corruption and redemption."
—*Kirkus* (starred review)
160 pp • $14.95 • 978-1-933372-18-1

The Fugitive
"[Carlotto is] the reigning king of Mediterranean noir."
—*The Boston Phoenix*
176 pp • $14.95 • 978-1-933372-25-9

Francisco Coloane
Tierra del Fuego
"Coloane is the Jack London of our times."—Alvaro Mutis
176 pp • $14.95 • 978-1-933372-63-1

Giancarlo De Cataldo
The Father and the Foreigner
"A slim but touching noir novel from one of Italy's best writers
in the genre."—*Quaderni Noir*
160 pp • $15.00 • 978-1-933372-72-3

Shashi Deshpande
The Dark Holds No Terrors
"[Deshpande is] an extremely talented storyteller."—*Hindustan Times*
272 pp • $15.00 • 978-1-933372-67-9

Steve Erickson
Zeroville
"A funny, disturbing, daring and demanding novel—Erickson's best."
—*The New York Times Book Review*
352 pp • $14.95 • 978-1-933372-39-6

Elena Ferrante
The Days of Abandonment
"The raging, torrential voice of [this] author is something rare."
—*The New York Times*
192 pp • $14.95 • 978-1-933372-00-6

Troubling Love
"Ferrante's polished language belies the rawness
of her imagery."—*The New Yorker*
144 pp • $14.95 • 978-1-933372-16-7

The Lost Daughter
"So refined, almost translucent."—*The Boston Globe*
144 pp • $14.95 • 978-1-933372-42-6

Jane Gardam
Old Filth
"Old Filth belongs in the Dickensian pantheon of memorable characters."—*The New York Times Book Review*
304 pp • $14.95 • 978-1-933372-13-6

The Queen of the Tambourine
"A truly superb and moving novel."—*The Boston Globe*
272 pp • $14.95 • 978-1-933372-36-5

The People on Privilege Hill
"Engrossing stories of hilarity and heartbreak."—*Seattle Times*
208 pp • $15.95 • 978-1-933372-56-3

Alicia Giménez-Bartlett
Dog Day
"Delicado and Garzón prove to be one of the more engaging sleuth teams to debut in a long time."—*The Washington Post*
320 pp • $14.95 • 978-1-933372-14-3

Prime Time Suspect
"A gripping police procedural."—*The Washington Post*
320 pp • $14.95 • 978-1-933372-31-0

Death Rites
"Petra is developing into a good cop, and her earnest efforts to assert her authority…are worth cheering."—*The New York Times*
304 pp • $16.95 • 978-1-933372-54-9

Katharina Hacker
The Have-Nots
"Hacker's prose soars."—*Publishers Weekly*
352 pp • $14.95 • 978-1-933372-41-9

Patrick Hamilton
Hangover Square
"Patrick Hamilton's novels are dark tunnels of misery, loneliness, deceit, and sexual obsession."—*New York Review of Books*
336 pp • $14.95 • 978-1-933372-06-8

James Hamilton-Paterson
Cooking with Fernet Branca
"Irresistible!"—*The Washington Post*
288 pp • $14.95 • 978-1-933372-01-3

Amazing Disgrace
"It's loads of fun, light and dazzling as a peacock feather."
—*New York Magazine*
352 pp • $14.95 • 978-1-933372-19-8

Rancid Pansies
"Campy comic saga about hack writer and self-styled 'culinary genius' Gerald Samper."—*Seattle Times*
288 pp • $15.95 • 978-1-933372-62-4

Seven-Tenths: The Sea and Its Thresholds
"The kind of book that, were he alive now, Shelley might have written."
—Charles Sprawson
416 pp • $16.00 • 978-1-933372-69-3

www.europaeditions.com

Alfred Hayes
The Girl on the Via Flaminia
"Immensely readable."—*The New York Times*
160 pp • $14.95 • 978-1-933372-24-2

Jean-Claude Izzo
Total Chaos
"Izzo's Marseilles is ravishing."—*Globe and Mail*
256 pp • $14.95 • 978-1-933372-04-4

Chourmo
"A bitter, sad and tender salute to a place equally impossible
to love or leave."—*Kirkus* (starred review)
256 pp • $14.95 • 978-1-933372-17-4

Solea
"[Izzo is] a talented writer who draws from the deep, dark well
of noir."—*The Washington Post*
208 pp • $14.95 • 978-1-933372-30-3

The Lost Sailors
"Izzo digs deep into what makes men weep."
—*Time Out New York*
272 pp • $14.95 • 978-1-933372-35-8

A Sun for the Dying
"Beautiful, like a black sun, tragic and desperate."—*Le Point*
224 pp • $15.00 • 978-1-933372-59-4

Gail Jones
Sorry
"Jones's gift for conjuring place and mood rarely falters."
—*Times Literary Supplement*
240 pp • $15.95 • 978-1-933372-55-6

Matthew F. Jones
Boot Tracks
"A gritty action tale."—*The Philadelphia Inquirer*
208 pp • $14.95 • 978-1-933372-11-2

Ioanna Karystiani
The Jasmine Isle
"A modern Greek tragedy about love foredoomed
and family life."—*Kirkus*
288 pp • $14.95 • 978-1-933372-10-5

Gene Kerrigan
The Midnight Choir
"The lethal precision of his closing punches leave quite a lasting mark."
—*Entertainment Weekly*
368 pp • $14.95 • 978-1-933372-26-6

Little Criminals
"A great story...relentless and brilliant."—Roddy Doyle
352 pp • $16.95 • 978-1-933372-43-3

Peter Kocan
Fresh Fields
"A stark, harrowing, yet deeply courageous work of immense power and magnitude."—*Quadrant*
304 pp • $14.95 • 978-1-933372-29-7

The Treatment and the Cure
"Kocan tells this story with grace and humor."—*Publishers Weekly*
256 pp • $15.95 • 978-1-933372-45-7

Helmut Krausser
Eros
"Helmut Krausser has succeeded in writing a great German epochal novel."—*Focus*
352 pp • $16.95 • 978-1-933372-58-7

Amara Lakhous
Clash of Civilizations Over an Elevator in Piazza Vittorio
"Do we have an Italian Camus on our hands? Just possibly."
—*The Philadelphia Inquirer*
144 pp • $14.95 • 978-1-933372-61-7

Carlo Lucarelli

Carte Blanche

"Lucarelli proves that the dark and sinister are better evoked when one opts for unadulterated grit and grime."
—*The San Diego Union-Tribune*
128 pp • $14.95 • 978-1-933372-15-0

The Damned Season

"De Luca…is a man both pursuing and pursued. And that makes him one of the more interesting figures in crime fiction."
—*The Philadelphia Inquirer*
128 pp • $14.95 • 978-1-933372-27-3

Via delle Oche

"Delivers a resolution true to the series' moral relativism."
—*Publishers Weekly*
160 pp • $14.95 • 978-1-933372-53-2

Edna Mazya

Love Burns

"Combines the suspense of a murder mystery with the absurdity of a Woody Allen movie."—*Kirkus*
224 pp • $14.95 • 978-1-933372-08-2

Sélim Nassib
I Loved You for Your Voice
"Nassib spins a rhapsodic narrative out of the indissoluble
connection between two creative souls."—*Kirkus*
272 pp • $14.95 • 978-1-933372-07-5

The Palestinian Lover
"A delicate, passionate novel in which history and life are
inextricably entwined."—*RAI Books*
192 pp • $14.95 • 978-1-933372-23-5

Amélie Nothomb
Tokyo Fiancée
"Intimate and honest…depicts perfectly a nontraditional romance."
—*Publishers Weekly*
160 pp • $15.00 • 978-1-933372-64-8

Alessandro Piperno
The Worst Intentions
"A coruscating mixture of satire, family epic, Proustian meditation,
and erotomaniacal farce."—*The New Yorker*
320 pp • $14.95 • 978-1-933372-33-4

Eric-Emmanuel Schmitt
The Most Beautiful Book in the World
"Nine novellas, parables on the idea of a future, filled with redeeming
optimism."—*Lire Magazine*
192 pp • $15.00 • 978-1-933372-74-7

Domenico Starnone
First Execution
"Starnone's books are small theatres of action, both physical
and psychological."—*L'espresso* (Italy)
176 pp • $15.00 • 978-1-933372-66-2

Joel Stone
The Jerusalem File
"Joel Stone is a major new talent."—*Cleveland Plain Dealer*
160 pp • $15.00 • 978-1-933372-65-5

Benjamin Tammuz
Minotaur
"A novel about the expectations and compromises that humans create
for themselves."—*The New York Times*
192 pp • $14.95 • 978-1-933372-02-0

Chad Taylor
Departure Lounge
"There's so much pleasure and bafflement to be derived
from this thriller."—*The Chicago Tribune*
176 pp • $14.95 • 978-1-933372-09-9

Roma Tearne
Mosquito
"Vividly rendered…Wholly satisfying."—*Kirkus*
352 pp • $16.95 • 978-1-933372-57-0

Bone China
"Tearne deftly reveals the corrosive effects of civil strife on private lives and the redemptiveness of art."—*The Guardian*
432 pp • $16.00 • 978-1-933372-75-4

Christa Wolf
One Day a Year: 1960-2000
"Remarkable!"—*The New Yorker*
640 pp • $16.95 • 978-1-933372-22-8

Edwin M. Yoder Jr.
Lions at Lamb House
"Yoder writes with such wonderful manners, learning, and detachment."—William F. Buckley, Jr.
256 pp • $14.95 • 978-1-933372-34-1

Michele Zackheim
Broken Colors
"A beautiful novel."—*Library Journal*
320 pp • $14.95 • 978-1-933372-37-2